OXFORD ANAESTHESIA LIBRARY

Anaesthesia for the Overweight and Obese Patient

Mark Bellamy

Professor of Critical Care Anaesthesia,
Department of Anaesthesia,
St. James's University Hospital,
Leeds, UK

Michel Struys

Professor in Anesthesia and Research Co-ordinator,
Department of Anesthesia, Ghent University Hospital,
Ghent, Belgium

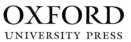

OXFORD
UNIVERSITY PRESS

OXFORD
UNIVERSITY PRESS

Great Clarendon Street, Oxford OX2 6DP

Oxford University Press is a department of the University of Oxford.
It furthers the University's objective of excellence in research, scholarship,
and education by publishing worldwide in

Oxford New York

Auckland Cape Town Dar es Salaam Hong Kong Karachi
Kuala Lumpur Madrid Melbourne Mexico City Nairobi
New Delhi Shanghai Taipei Toronto

With offices in

Argentina Austria Brazil Chile Czech Republic France Greece
Guatemala Hungary Italy Japan Poland Portugal Singapore
South Korea Switzerland Thailand Turkey Ukraine Vietnam

Oxford is a registered trade mark of Oxford University Press
in the UK and in certain other countries

Published in the United States
by Oxford University Press Inc., New York

British Library Cataloguing in Publication Data

Data available

Library of Congress Cataloging in Publication Data

Data available

Typeset by Newgen Imaging Systems (P) Ltd., Chennai, India
Printed in China
on acid-free paper by
Phoenix Offset Ltd

ISBN 978-0-19-923395-3

10 9 8 7 6 5 4 3 2 1

Whilst every effort has been made to ensure that the contents of this book are as
complete, accurate and-up-to-date as possible at the date of writing. Oxford
University Press is not able to give any guarantee or assurance that such is the case.
Readers are urged to take appropriately qualified medical advice in all cases. The
information in this book is intended to be useful to the general reader, but should
not be used as a means of self-diagnosis or for the prescription of medication.

Contents

vi

Preface

Introduction

Obesity is a major health care challenge for the Western world. It has been a problem in the United States for many years. Healthcare trends in Western Europe tend to follow those in the United States, around 10 years later. The World Health Organisation recently reported that both childhood and adult obesity have increased dramatically in prevalence in Western Europe in recent years. Childhood obesity is now 10 times more common than it was in 1970.

In the adult population, 50% are overweight, and one third are obese. This has huge implications for health care costs as well as for the economy at large. In the Western Europe, 6% of health care expenditure is attributable to obesity, and this figure is set to rise dramatically.

Morbidly obese patients suffer numerous comorbidities. This presents a huge challenge to the anaesthetist. While raised BMI is not of itself a predictor of poor postoperative outcome, obesity related comorbidity is a strong predictor, and is very common. Moreover, the morbidly obese and super obese patient poses considerable technical challenges to the anaesthetist. Over 50% of critical incidents reported in anaesthesia involve obesity as a contributory factor.

This book is aimed at the general anaesthetist who is likely to encounter increasingly large numbers of morbidly obese and super obese patients in his everyday practice over the next few years. Morbidly obese patients present for elective surgery for unrelated conditions, for procedures related to obesity (including joint replacement or bariatric surgery) and for procedures related to their comorbidity (for example, vascular disease secondary to diabetes). In this book, we have aimed to outline the basics of obesity physiology and pathology, in the hope that this will give the anaesthetist and necessary building blocks with which to solve complex clinical problems. Additionally, we have given a number of practical hints and suggestions, based on our experience of anaesthesia for morbidly obese and super obese patients. While this experience has largely been derived from bariatric surgical practice, much of it is generalisable to other operative situations where morbidly obese patients are encountered.

Each chapter is followed by a further reading section, rather than an exhaustive reference list. The literature on obesity surgery, obesity comorbidities and anaesthesia for the obese is enlarging on an almost daily basis. While we have made every effort to ensure the text is based on the latest knowledge, the field is advancing so rapidly that we strongly recommend the interested reader to use this book as a starting point, and not as a definitive guide.

The authors are extremely grateful to those colleagues who have contributed to our clinical experience, and to those who have made helpful suggestions on the manuscript of this book. In particular, we are grateful to Professor Chris Dodds, director of the South Tees sleep laboratory, and to Mr Stephen Pollard, obesity surgeon, Leeds.

Mark C. Bellamy, Leeds, UK
Michel M.R.F. Struys, Ghent, Belgium
February 2007.

Further Reading

European Ministerial Conference on Counteracting Obesity. World Health Organisation. Istanbul. 2007.
http://www.euro.who.int/Document/E89567.pdf

Chapter 1

Definitions, social trends, and epidemiology

Key points

- Obesity is an epidemic facing society at large.
- Body mass index is widely used to define obesity but waist circumference is more predictive of morbidity.
- Obese >30 kg per square metre.
- Morbidly obese >40 kg per square metre.
- 43% of men and 33% of women are overweight.
- 22% of men and 23% of women are obese.
- In the United Kingdom, obesity results in 30,000 deaths per year.
- The estimated cost to the National Health Service in the United Kingdom is between £0.5 and £1 billion annually.
- When the obese patient presents for anaesthesia, the challenges to the anaesthetist and theatre team are very real.

1.1 Obesity: the size of the problem

Obesity is an epidemic facing society at large. It is a challenge to all health care professionals. The problems faced by the anaesthetist are different from those facing other health care professionals: whereas many doctors and other carers have to deal with the root causes of obesity, or its complications, the anaesthetist is faced with treating the patient for intercurrent disease. Often, this means providing anaesthesia for a condition completely unrelated to obesity or its co-morbidities. Nevertheless, the presence of these co-morbidities may result in increased difficulty for the anaesthetist and greatly increased risk for the patient. Moreover, obesity is characterised by anatomical and physiological changes, which may provide challenges of a very mundane and practical nature for the anaesthetist, surgeon, and other theatre staff. These may be extremely difficult to deal with.

Awareness of the issues, together with advanced planning, can go a long way to meeting these challenges, but does not completely obviate them.

The rising prevalence of overweight and obesity in the UK population is part of a worldwide obesity pandemic. In the United States, the problem runs about 10 years ahead of that in Europe. It is estimated that between 40 and 50 million Americans are obese. This means that many of the issues which we are facing now have already been faced by our colleagues in the United States for a number of years. Some solutions have been reached; however, the changes in culture and resource provision available to the doctor in the United States in many cases have not yet reached Europe. A number of definitions have been used to quantify this problem, and these definitions will be used in this book.

1.2 Body mass index

The body mass index (BMI) is the most widely used measurement and has become the standard by which the body habitus of a patient is described. Although BMI is not the best clinical predictor of much co-morbidity (simple measurements such as waist circumference and neck circumference are often better), it is nevertheless the common currency of measurement and has become universally adopted. The BMI is calculated by dividing the weight of the patient (expressed in kilograms) by the square of the patient's height (expressed in metres and decimals of a metre). The resulting figure is the BMI (Table 1.1). Values below 20 kg per square metre represent under weight. Between 20 and 25 represents ideal body weight. Up to 30 kg per square metre is considered overweight and above 30 is described as obese. 'Morbid obesity' relates to those individuals who have a BMI greater than 40. In some definitions, morbid obesity also includes those with a BMI above 35, but who have already developed obesity-related co-morbidities, such as type 2 diabetes, obstructive sleep apnoea, etc.

As weight increases further, there is a higher prevalence of obesity-related co-morbidities, and of problems directly related to weight, anatomical change, and physiological change. The term 'super obese' is used to describe those with a BMI greater than 50 kg per square metre, and the term 'super super obese' is used to describe those with a BMI of greater than 60. Individuals with a BMI greater than 70 were historically very rare, but are now seen increasingly frequently in clinical practice. This group is sometimes called 'hyper obese'.

Table 1.1 Definitions of obesity by body mass index (BMI)	
BMI (kgm⁻²)	Descriptor
<20	Underweight
20–24.9	Ideal
25–29.9	Overweight
30–39.9	Obese
40–49.9 or 35–49.9 with obesity-related co-morbidity	Morbidly obese
50–59.9	Super obese
60–69.9	Super super obese
>70	Hyper obese

The BMI is however not a perfect tool. As mentioned earlier, a number of other measures, such as girth measurement, are often more predictive of clinical sequelae. The BMI is a somewhat blunt tool. For example, clinical consequences relate not only to the 'size' of the lesion (as estimated by BMI) but also to the duration of the obesity and age of the patient. Further, BMI is most useful only in patients with a typical body habitus whose height is around the middle of the normal range. The BMI tends to overestimate obesity in tall subjects and in muscular subjects. At the same time, it underestimates the size of the lesion in shorter subjects.

BMI likewise fails to take account of fat distribution. This is why simple linear measurements such as girth or neck circumference are often more clinically valuable. There is a spectrum of types of fat distribution; most individuals will lie somewhere on this spectrum, although some have an entirely unique fat distribution. So to some extent, every individual is different! Nevertheless, there are two major types classified. In the android fat distribution most of the weight is carried on the trunk, and there is a high intra-peritoneal fat content. The patient is often heavy jowled, with an increased neck circumference, but the arms and legs are relatively spared. In contrast, the patient with a gynaecoid fat distribution tends to have excess fat in the arms, legs, and buttocks. The head and neck are often relatively spared. In the gynaecoid fat distribution, abdominal fat is predominantly extra peritoneal.

Other measures of body mass are also used in clinical practice – for example, when estimating drug doses. Total body weight, ideal body weight, and lean body weight are all useful in clinical practice.

1.3 **Trends in obesity**

Health researchers, public health physicians, economists, and health care planners are becoming increasingly concerned about the size and rapid growth of the obesity pandemic. There is a clear concern regarding both health care provision and cost implications of obesity. The Department of Health (England and Wales) has commissioned several reports into the subject. These studies have confirmed clinical impression. Since 1993, the average weight of the population has measurably increased. In the teenage boys and girls, for example, the mean BMI has risen by around 1 kg per square metre in the 10-year period following 1993. This figure, however, masks the size of the problem overall.

According to a 2001 report, the National Audit Office for England classified 43% of men and 29% of women as overweight, and 13% of men and 16% of women were classified as obese. In 2006, the Department of Health commissioned a further report to assess the current position, and estimate accurately the size of the obesity problem by 2010. This report revised the figures substantially upwards: although the number of overweight men had changed little since 1993, the number of overweight women had risen to 33%, and the number of *obese* men and women had risen to 22 and 23%, respectively. Worryingly, there was also a substantial increase in obesity in children (as assessed by the number of children whose weights were above traditional 85% centile values).

The report concluded that there were clear trends in obesity. Although the number of overweight individuals had not changed much since 1993, the number of obese individuals had. This suggests that an entire section of the population had gained weight spectacularly, while other sections of the population had maintained a BMI close to traditional values. For every overweight patient who has progressed to become obese, an 'ideal weight' patient had progressed to being overweight. Not all groups in society had behaved in an equivalent manner. For example, the increase in overweight and obesity has been greatest in the Midlands and North of England, and least in London and the southeast. The increase in weight in men was slightly greater in manual workers as compared with office workers, whereas in women there was a much greater increase in those with sedentary occupations as compared with manual workers. Finally, current trends suggest a greater increase in the prevalence of overweight and obesity in the white than in the non-white population (although the problem is seen to some extent across all social and racial groups). This is offset by the fact that co-morbidity and obesity-related medical problems such as diabetes seem to have very high levels in Middle Eastern and South Asian populations, so a slightly lower prevalence of obesity does not necessarily translate to a lower prevalence of obesity-related co-morbidities.

1.4 **Health and economic costs**

Many commentators have noted that, in terms of health care provision, we have a very limited time to act. This is because the existing level of overweight and obesity in the population, particularly in the young population, represents a health care 'time bomb'. Those who are obese now are already at risk, and although they (in most cases) have not yet developed obesity-related co-morbidities, many will do so. In particular, the number of cases of type 2 diabetes is likely to increase explosively over the next 10–20 years. This will be the legacy of existing levels of obesity. The situation is compounded by the fact that obesity is not constant at present levels; there is no indication the obesity pandemic is slowing.

The economy at large suffers both directly and indirectly from the costs of obesity. It has been estimated that in the United Kingdom, obesity results in 30,000 deaths per year, equating to nine lost years of life in afflicted individuals. These figures rival those for carcinoma of the breast. The estimated cost to the National Health Service in the United Kingdom is between £0.5 and 1 billion annually. Obesity accounts for 18 million days of sick leave each year, with a cost to the wider economy has been estimated at between £2 and 3.5 billion each year. The situation in many other European countries is very similar.

The health care consequences of obesity are far reaching. A number of strategies have been suggested to deal with them. First, we can try to cope with the 'fallout' of the problem. This would entail treating the ill-health resulting from obesity and its various co-morbidities, and represents a default position. Clearly, this is not a desirable long-term option, as there is an ever-increasing prevalence of obesity-related co-morbidity in the community.

Second, potentially huge benefits could accrue from even modest weight reduction in the general population. By treating obesity in the ever-growing number of affected individuals, by dietary help, health care advice, exercise programs, specific treatments (including drug therapies, and as a last resort, surgery), it is possible to prevent the evolution of co-morbidities and their complications.

Third, it has been suggested that it may be possible to reduce the social and economic trends which have contributed to the explosion in obesity. Obesity and its problems, while they may affect individuals who are economically deprived, are not general problems found in societies facing economic hardship. Such societal changes tend to arise independently of the wilful intentions of society leaders, and are certainly beyond the scope of anaesthetic practice!

1.5 **Obesity and the anaesthetist**

The anaesthetist is likely to encounter obese subjects in several arenas. First, an increasing number of obese patients present for surgery on general operating lists, either for problems related to obesity (for example, orthopaedic surgery, cancer surgery) or for completely unrelated problems. Second, there are those patients who present acutely out of hours for emergency surgery. In many ways, this is the more challenging group, as they are generally less well prepared and poorly investigated compared with the elective patient. Moreover, they may present to a theatre team with relatively little experience of the very obese patient, or in a situation where appropriate expertise, advice, or equipment is hard to come by.

Third, the morbidly obese patient may present for weight reduction surgery. This represents in some ways the easiest situation; as such, patients have the opportunity for full assessment and investigation. They enjoy the benefit of being treated by individuals with considerable experience and presumably expertise in the care of patients with morbid obesity. They further enjoy the benefits of a suitable environment, including adequately staffed operating theatres, which are appropriately equipped for the obese subject. Finally, their surgery can be deferred if either the peri-operative environment or the post-operative resource is less than ideal. Against this, they tend to be patients with the highest BMIs, and greatest prevalence and severity of obesity-related complications.

Whatever the circumstances and setting in which the obese patient presents for anaesthesia, the challenges to the anaesthetist and theatre team are very real. Such challenges are likely to become more frequent and more difficult over the next few years.

Further reading

Haslam D, Sattar N, Lean M. (2006) Obesity – time to wake up. *Br Med J* **333**: 640–2.

National Audit Office. Tackling Obesity in England. London: NAO, 2001. http://www.nao.org.uk/pn/00-01/0001220.htm

Zaninotto P, Wardle H, Stamatakis E, Mindell J, Head J. (2006). Forecasting Obesity to 2010. London: National Centre for Social Research, http://www.dh.gov.uk/assetRoot/04/13/86/29/04138629.pdf

Chapter 2

Physiology of obesity, molecular, and medical approaches

Key points

- Many overweight and obese people have an extremely negative body image.
- Poor body image may contribute to the persistence of obesity.
- Reduction in activity and increased calorie consumption are obligatory consequences of obesity, not simply causes of obesity.
- The pathways of energy balance represent a three limb process, orchestrated by the hypothalamus.
- There is probably a strong individual genetic component, with everyone having their own 'leptin set point'.
- Medical strategies include behaviour and lifestyle modification, and drug therapy.
- The contribution of pharmacological therapy is limited.

2.1 General considerations

Obese subjects are common in society. Obesity frequently attracts prejudice, and indeed negative remarks. Many of the prejudices that we hold our subliminal, but exist nonetheless. They are readily demonstrated by the psychological experiments. Prejudice against obese individuals is often subtle, but affects their opportunities, self-image, and lifestyle.

Negative views regarding overweight and obese individuals are shared by those people themselves, and in many cases intensely so. Many overweight and obese people have an extremely negative body image that is severely debilitating. This frequently limits lifestyle, and social and economic opportunities. This problem is particularly severe in young people, and can serve to constrain activity as much as physical manifestations of obesity. In children, this has been reported as causing a reduction in quality-of-life comparable to the distress of undergoing cancer chemotherapy. The vicious cycle of shyness, social disadvantage, and psychological defence mechanisms, such as staying indoors, lack of exercise, overeating, and continuing poor body image, at least contribute to the persistence of obesity in some cases, but they clearly represent an incomplete picture in many individuals.

There has historically been a view that the cause of obesity is over-eating in combination with inadequate exercise. This is a simple view and a very attractive one. It possesses the elegance of simplicity and seems to accord well with the basic laws of physics. Despite the elegance of the argument, there are flaws and exceptions, which have led us to re-evaluate this simple position. For example, there are some people who seem to remain the same irrespective of how much they eat. They do not seem to exercise frequently, strenuously come up, or any more than other people who weigh much more. Others seem to eat relatively little, but to gain weight easily. Those who gain weight do not all gain it according to the same weight distribution. Of those who become overweight and obese, not all shown the same physiological deterioration, all developed the same at range, or severity of co-morbidities. These and other observations suggest that the situation is far more complex than a simple energy balance equation.

Current approaches to the pathology of obesity turn the energy balance equation on its head. It seems very likely that in most cases, the reduction in activity and increased calorie consumption are obligatory consequences of obesity, resulting from underlying genetic and hormonal changes, and cannot simply be viewed as primary causes of obesity within the control of the patient.

A number of pathways are thought to be involved in these interactions. These have not all been clearly elucidated and many features are poorly understood. Most models contain common key features. These include hyperinsulinaemia (leading to increased deposition of fat), insulin resistance (associated with type 2 diabetes), suppressed or defective leptin signal transduction (resulting in reduced satiety), and an insulin-mediated reduction in dopamine clearance in the primitive parts of the brain, resulting in an increased 'food reward'.

These factors taken together mean that the physiological changes of obesity, which may result from a combination of genetic factors and environmental opportunity, may result in an obligate increase in caloric consumption and reduction in fat utilisation. Thus, in many patients, treatment may need to be aimed at not only breaking but also permanently suppressing this vicious circle. This is difficult because of the complex and robust nature of the pathways involved in auto regulation of adiposity and satiety.

2.2 **Pathways of energy balance**

The pathways of energy balance represent a three limb process, orchestrated by the hypothalamus. The afferent limb involves peripheral signalling to the central nervous system. The ventromedial hypothalamus receives signalling from leptin (adipose tissue content), central nervous signalling effects of insulin (acute metabolic status), ghrelin (from the stomach signalling hunger), and peptide YY_{3-36} (from the small intestine signalling satiety).

These signals are integrated in the hypothalamus, together with inputs from other parts of the central nervous system. The second limb of the process signals these inputs to the paraventricular nucleus of the hypothalamus and the lateral hypothalamic area. Occupancy of the melanocortin 4 receptor integrates these to regulate energy balance. These signals either reduce the appetite (*anorexigenic*, for example, alpha melanocyte-stimulating hormone) or increase it (*orexigenic*, for example, neuropeptide Y).

The efferent limb of the reflex arc is mediated predominantly through the autonomic nervous system. The sympathetic nervous system is responsible for increased energy use, and the parasympathetic nervous system (vagal stimulation) is involved in insulin secretion and energy storage. Insulin is part of the efferent pathway (as an effector) as well as part of the afferent pathway as a transducing signal.

2.3 **Leptin**

Leptin is a hormone released from the adipose tissue. It signals adipose tissue mass, and hence adequacy of the energy supply, to the central nervous system. Through its role in the reflex arc described above, leptin increases melanocyte-stimulating hormone and inhibits neuropeptide Y. Overall, therefore, its effect is to reduce food intake and permit increased energy expenditure.

2.4 **Insulin**

Aside from its well-known role as an effector in this system (peripheral effects), insulin has an important role as a signal to the central nervous system as part of the afferent limb of the energy balance pathway. These central nervous system effects of insulin are similar to those of leptin. Indeed, the central nervous system insulin receptors are localised in the same neurones in the ventromedial hypothalamus. Insulin access the central nervous system via a specific transporter. In increased levels of insulin within the central nervous system reduce feeding and cause satiety. They activate the sympathetic nervous system by a mechanism similar to that resulting from increased leptin levels. Indeed, it is thought that insulin and leptin share a common second messenger system.

2.5 **Sympathetic nervous system**

In response to signalling by insulin and leptin, there is increased activity in the sympathetic nervous system. In experimental animals, this results in an increase in thermogenesis and breakdown of brown fat, together with increased levels of motor activity. Sympathetic stimulation in man results in increased energy expenditure through glycogen breakdown, and through oxidation of glucose and fatty acids in skeletal muscle. It further results in adipose tissue lipolysis. These effects are mediated by the beta 3 adrenergic receptor, by increasing both the expression and activity of uncoupling proteins, and through hormone-sensitive lipase.

2.6 **Parasympathetic nervous system**

The effects of the parasympathetic nervous system, and in particular, the vagus nerve, oppose those of the sympathetic nervous system. Stimulation of the vagus nerve modulates beta cell function in the pancreas and results in increased secretion of insulin. This in turn results in an increased deposition of energy substrates into fatty tissue. In animal models, the vagus nerve also synapses on adipose cells and increases the insulin sensitivity of these cells. It is not known whether this also occurs in man.

2.7 **Starvation and the leptin set point**

Appetite and obesity seem to be regulated in different individuals according to a 'leptin set point'. It has been postulated that this is genetically determined. During dieting or starvation (similar effects are seen with weight reduction medications), there is an initial reduction in weight. In parallel with the fall in the adipose tissue mass, there is a reduction in leptin levels. Even if dietary medications are continued, or the dietary calorie intake is maintained at a low level, weight reduction does not continue beyond about four months. This was previously attributed to non-compliance or drug tolerance. More recent works have shown that reduced leptin levels result in a 'starvation response', in which there is a reduction of around 20% in resting energy expenditure. This reduction in resting energy expenditure balances the reduced calorie intake, so that weight loss is not sustained. This can be seen even in short-term fasting and starvation, where an acute reduction in leptin results in a hypothalamus-mediated increase in vagal tone and a reduction in sympathetic stimulation. Interestingly, both leptin-deficient humans and knockout mice exhibit behavioural and biochemical manifestations of a chronic starvation response.

At least two forms of central nervous system lesion have been characterised in which the hypothalamic response to leptin is lost. These include 'idiopathic obesity', in which there is functional leptin resistance, and 'hypothalamic obesity', where hypothalamic damage leads to organic leptin resistance. Hypothalamic obesity is remarkably resistant to medical therapies, changes in diet, or behaviour.

Although the acute central nervous system responses to leptin and insulin are similar, insulin is more responsible for short-term changes and leptin signals for longer-term (body habitus) changes. In obesity, there is a loss of negative feedback response, which would normally occur as a consequence of leptin or insulin exposure. As a result of this, high levels of insulin or leptin do not result in satiety, and sympathetic stimulation (and, therefore, thermogenesis and resting energy expenditure) remain low. Moreover, chronically high insulin levels have been described as antagonising leptin signalling.

2.8 **Food reward pathways**

In addition to their direct effects on orexia and anorexia, insulin and leptin also modify the pleasure response to eating. These are mediated in the ventral tegmental area and the nucleus accumbens. The response to eating, in common with that to drugs of addiction, is mediated by an increase in dopamine release and its action on dopamine D2 receptors. In animal models, both insulin and dopamine receptor antagonists act in an additive way to reduce the reward response to eating. It is thought that insulin resistance in the ventral tegmental area is a possible cause of obesity by facilitating dopamine accumulation in the nucleus accumbens, hence enhancing the pleasure response to food.

2.9 **Medical approaches to the management of obesity**

An increasing number of obese patients seek medical help in an attempt to tackle this problem. Medical therapy is aimed at

- weight loss
- weight maintenance (6 months or more)
- reduction in risk factors.

Medical strategies include behaviour and lifestyle modification, and drug therapy. Behavioural modification focuses on regular exercise, an increase in energy expenditure, sensible eating, and dietary advice.

These strategies tend to be ineffective by themselves, and so are often supported by exercises such as maintaining a diary or attending support groups. There are many web-based self-help and support groups, as well as a large 'slimming industry'. Despite this, many individuals still struggle.

A reduction in dietary calorie intake of 600 kcal a day results in a weight reduction of around 5 kg at 1 year, falling to between 2 and 4 kg at 3 years. Dramatically, the effect of adding exercise to diet is a modest weight loss of around 2 kg at 1 year, but a major weight loss of 8 kg at 3 years. The United Kingdom Department of Health has published recommendations on physical activity for adults (Table 2.1). The majority of obese subjects are thought to exercise less than the recommendations.

Table 2.1 Department of health recommendations on physical activity for adults
30 min of at least moderate activity on at least 5 days a week
For many people, 45–60 min of moderate activity a day may be necessary to prevent obesity
People who have been obese and have managed to lose weight may need to do 60–90 min of activity daily to maintain weight loss
Recommended levels of activity may be obtained in one session or as bouts of activity of 10 min or more
The activity can be 'lifestyle' activity (such as walking, cycling, climbing stairs, hoovering, mowing lawn), structured exercise, or sport http://www.dh.gov.uk/assetRoot/04/08/09/88/04080988.pdf

2.10 **Drug therapies**

Many obese patients also undergo drug therapy to aid weight reduction or to reduce the risk of co-morbidity. Again, the basic principles are weight loss, weight maintenance, and reduction of other risk factors. As the origin of obesity is multifactorial, the contribution of pharmacological therapy is limited. After stopping the medication, a rebound phenomenon has been described. Although beneficial effects on the cardiovascular risk factor have been found, no outcome data on morbidity and mortality are available. Most of the drugs have side effects.

The main drugs currently used for the management of obesity are as follows.

2.10.1 **Sibutramine**

This drug acts in the central nervous system to enhance and prolong satiety. It inhibits the re-uptake of noradrenaline and serotonin. A once daily dose is said to produce weight loss of 5–10% in majority of the patients. It is relatively well tolerated in most cases. Some patients find anti-cholinergic side effects troublesome. Sleep disturbance may also be a feature. Those patients who fail to lose weight may occasionally become hypertensive while taking sibutramine. Again, this mandates close observation of such patients, and limits the usefulness of the drug.

2.10.2 **Orlistat**

This drug is taken three times daily with food, and acts as a lipase inhibitor in the intestine. It results in malabsorption of up to 30% of ingested fat. Again, this results in a weight loss of around 5–10% in the majority of patients. This weight loss can be maintained for several years. It is associated with an improvement in the risk factors for coronary heart disease and diabetes. There may be a secondary effect on improving insulin sensitivity. Side effects include steatorrhoea in patients who fail to adhere to a low-fat diet. There is no clinical evidence for combining treatments with orlistat and sibutramine.

2.10.3 **Rimonabant**

This is a novel cannabinoid-1 receptor antagonist. It is thought to act by reducing the reward response to eating in the ventral tegmental area and the nucleus accumbens. In common with other medications, it produces a 5–10% weight loss and concomitant but apparently independent improvements in cardiovascular risk factors. Clinical trials have suggested that the drug is well tolerated, although there may be effects on factor. The drug is avoided in depressed patients.

2.11 **Conclusions**

The pathways involved in the regulation of appetite and fat metabolism are complex. There is probably a strong individual genetic component, with everyone having their own 'leptin set point'. This results in a tendency towards constant adipose tissue mass independent of changes in diet. Central nervous system sensitivity to insulin is central to modulating the reward response to food as well as short-term autonomic nervous system responses. Combined dietary, behavioural, and exercise strategies produce the greatest (more than additive) changes in adipose tissue content and obesity. This could be because a combined strategy interrupts the physiological feedback loop responsible for the tendency towards a constant whole-body adipose tissue mass.

Many obese patients are taking medical therapies to manage their obesity or its complications. These therapies may have important implications for central nervous system performance and cardiovascular function in the perioperative period.

Further reading

Lean M, Finer N (2006). ABC of obesity. Management: Part II – Drugs. *Br Med J* **333**: 794–7.

Lustig RH (2001). The neuroendocrinology of childhood obesity. *Pediatr Clin North Am* **48**: 909–30.

Lustig RH (2006). Childhood obesity: behavioral aberration or biochemical drive? Reinterpreting the First Law of Thermodynamics. *Nat Clin Pract* **2**(8): 447–58.

Chapter 3

Obesity and systemic physiology

Key points

- Obesity and related co-morbidities result in physiological abnormalities that can have a major impact in the perioperative period.
- Not all features of physiological derangement are seen in all patients.
- Gynaecoid fat distribution is less severe, whereas the android fat distribution carries greater pathophysiological significance.
- Both obstructive sleep apnoea and the obesity hypoventilation syndrome can result in a chronically raised carbon dioxide tension.
- As body mass index increases, there is a progressive decline in functional residual capacity.
- There is an increased shunt in obese patients undergoing anaesthesia.
- The extent and severity of cardiovascular changes seen in obesity is highly variable, depending on factors including body mass index and duration of obesity.
- Increase in body mass index results in increased myocardial fat content and reduced contractility.
- Many obese patients develop right heart complications.
- The prevalence of fatty liver is up to 90%.
- Hiatus hernia is common in morbid obesity.

The interrelationship between abnormal physiology and obesity is a complex one. Deranged physiology both at molecular and systemic level contributes to the development of obesity, and may determine the severity of its associated co-morbidities. In turn, both obesity and related co-morbidities result in physiological abnormalities, which can have a major impact in the perioperative period. Some of the features of physiological derangement are obligate, whereas other elements arise according to the severity or duration of obesity. Not all features of physiological derangement are seen in all patients. Both environmental and genetic factors modify the development of abnormal physiology.

An appreciation of the spectrum of physiological changes is important at the time of pre-operative assessment as well as during subsequent anaesthesia. Not all features of alter physiology may be immediately apparent on clinical examination, and may need to be elicited by special investigations. Although some of the physiological changes are subtle and of relatively little clinical impact, others have a dramatic bearing on both the conduct of anaesthesia, the clinical course, and the outcome.

3.1 **Fat distribution**

Fat distribution has a significant bearing on the presence of other physiological disturbances. The gynaecoid fat distribution is less severe of the two major types, while the android fat distribution carries greater pathophysiological significance. In the gynaecoid fat distribution, there is preponderance towards peripheral distribution of fat (arms, legs, and buttocks), while in the android fat distribution there is a tendency towards greater central obesity, often with peripheral sparing. The android fat distribution is also associated with greater myocardial fat content, and a higher prevalence of cardiovascular disease and other complications. In men, the cut point defining these two distributions is a waist-to-hip ratio of 1.0. In women, the ratio defining the transition between the two fat distributions is 0.8. The android and gynaecoid distributions are sometimes described as 'apples and pears' because of the typical torso morphology (Figure 3.1).

These definitions are unnecessarily somewhat arbitrary. Some individuals may technically fall into one distribution, while displaying significant features of the other. Confounding factors include the presence of a large abdominal fat pannus. Although this often represents extra peritoneal fat, consistent with the gynaecoid fat distribution, it nevertheless increases the waist-to-hip ratio. Some patients have a fat distribution which renders classification; therefore, estimation of systemic physiological derangement becomes very difficult (Figure 3.2).

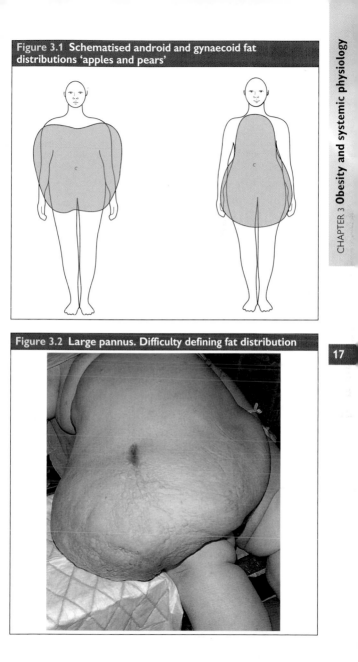

Figure 3.1 Schematised android and gynaecoid fat distributions 'apples and pears'

Figure 3.2 Large pannus. Difficulty defining fat distribution

3.2 **Respiratory system**

3.2.1 **Systemic effects**

Changes in the respiratory system can be subdivided into systemic changes, which affect 'respiration', in the sense of altered metabolism; and pulmonary changes, which predominantly affect gas exchange.

The basal metabolic rate of obese subjects is generally between 80 and 100% that of non-obese subjects. These values, however, are appropriate to the size of the individual. Most studies have quoted metabolic rates either relative to body weight or to body surface area. Compared with non-obese individuals, the absolute values of energy turnover are therefore significantly greater. This has several implications. First, obese individuals have a greater caloric expenditure. Second, and consequent on this, they have a greater caloric requirement to remain in the balance. Third, they have greater absolute oxygen consumption than non-obese subjects; and fourth, they have a greater absolute carbon dioxide production.

The absolute increase in oxygen consumption and carbon dioxide production have direct relevance to the delivery of anaesthesia, and particularly to oxygen requirements and therefore to fresh gas flows. This is of particular importance where low flow or closed circuit anaesthesia is used. The increased carbon dioxide production may mandate greater minute volumes to achieve normocapnea. Whether or not it is appropriate to achieve normocapnea is in itself debatable. Although it may be desirable in some clinical situations, there are others where correcting of the carbon dioxide tension to population that normal values represent a physiological abnormality for the individual patient.

Both obstructive sleep apnoea and the obesity hypoventilation syndrome can result in a chronically raised carbon dioxide tension. This results in renal retention of bicarbonate to maintain a normal pH. In turn, there is a relatively reduced alveolar minute volume and a reduced work of breathing. Although on the one hand this concerns energy expenditure, on the other hand it may contribute to a reduced tissue oxygen tension.

If such a patient is acutely ventilated to normocapnea, then a respiratory alkalosis results. Weaning from ventilation may thus be rendered difficult or impossible. Conversely, if 'normocapnea' is maintained by artificial ventilation for a prolonged period (e.g., in the intensive care setting or when a patient is ventilated for a very prolonged time in the operation theatre), then there may be sufficient time for renal adaptation to occur. This results in the excretion of bicarbonate and a consequent resetting of respiratory drive. In order to maintain a normal blood pH, when the patient is weaned from the ventilator, he/she has to achieve a lower arterial carbon dioxide tension. This implies a greater alveolar minute volume and an increased work of breathing. In severe cases, this can precipitate respiratory failure.

Moreover, patients who are chronically hypercarbic are likely to exhibit reduced sensitivity to a raised carbon dioxide tension. During anaesthesia, and in the perioperative period, this situation is exacerbated by the effects of anaesthetic drugs (and in particular, the volatile agents) as well as by opioid analgesics. All volatile agents have been described as reducing sensitivity to carbon dioxide even at very low volatile agent concentrations, and so the consequent effect of respiratory depression can be seen well into the post-anaesthetic recovery period (shown graphically in Figure 3.3).

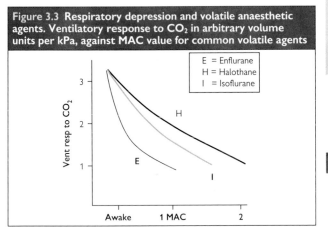

Figure 3.3 Respiratory depression and volatile anaesthetic agents. Ventilatory response to CO_2 in arbitrary volume units per kPa, against MAC value for common volatile agents

E = Enflurane
H = Halothane
I = Isoflurane

Vent resp to CO_2

Awake   1 MAC   2

3.2.2 **Pulmonary effects**
There is a clear relationship between increasing body mass index and pulmonary dysfunction. As body mass index increases, there is a progressive decline in functional residual capacity (FRC). In the normal and overweight ranges (up to a body mass index of 30 kgm^{-2}) in young adults, there is a progressive and steep reduction in FRC. However, this still exceeds 1 L. At a body mass index between 30 and 40 kgm^{-2}, FRC is typically less than 1 L, but the further reduction in FRC observed as body mass index increases beyond this follows a much gentler decline. It is not clear from the published data whether the reduction ever 'bottoms out'.

As body mass index increases, there is a similar fall in vital capacity and an increase in the alveolar to arterial oxygen tension gradient. In ventilated patients under anaesthesia, the change in alveolar to arterial oxygen tension gradient is a straight-line effect. It does not seem to attenuate at higher body mass indices. At a body mass index around 20 kgm^{-2}, the oxygen tension gradient is of the order of 7 kPa, rising steeply to a value around 25 kPa for patients with a body mass index of 70 kgm^{-2}.

Additionally, there is an increased shunt in obese patients undergoing anaesthesia. This is in part due to the effects of raised intra-abdominal pressure pushing upwards on the diaphragms and lung bases, together with the effects of a heavy chest wall compressing other regions of the lung. This enhanced airway closure combines with the effects of reduced FRC, resulting in substantial overlap between tidal volume breathing and closing volume during respiration or ventilation. The severity of this is in part related to factors such as fat distribution and intra-abdominal pressure. Hence, it is more severe in subjects with an android fat distribution. Airway closure and shunt may be further exacerbated by pre-existing airway collapse and atelectasis, especially in patients with obstructive sleep apnoea or where airway obstruction occurs during induction of anaesthesia.

The problems of airway closure are further compounded by a whole-body redistribution of circulating volume. This results in a return of circulating volume and pooling of blood in the central circulation, with a further increase in intra-pulmonary shunting.

In obesity, there is an increased work of breathing compared with normal subjects. This relates predominantly to reduced chest wall compliance. A consequence of this is the ease with which spontaneously breathing subjects can progress towards relative respiratory failure under (or subsequent to) anaesthesia. Conversely, ventilated subjects may require increased airway pressures relative to the non-obese to achieve similar tidal volume ventilation.

Positive end-inspiratory pressure is useful to prevent progressive airway de-recruitment. Sequential airway opening and closure is undesirable because of the theoretical risk of a bio transduction and generation of an inflammatory response. It is also likely that sequential airway opening and closure results overall in progressive airway collapse, and increases sheer forces between open and closed airway units, with a risk of volutrauma.

A recent work has suggested that much of the atelectasis and airway collapse seen during anaesthesia for morbidly obese subjects occurs in the period immediately following induction of anaesthesia. In bariatric surgery, a recruitment manoeuvre performed at this stage can provide airway opening and improvements in oxygenation, which are sustained throughout the remainder of the operative period. Also, the use of continuous positive airway pressure (CPAP) during induction might help to prevent atelactasis. Further, avoiding an F_iO_2 of 1.0 before intubation might protect against atelactasis formation.

3.3 **Functional respiratory effects**

Obesity interacts both with drugs and with site of surgery to produce reductions in vital capacity and oxygenation. There is a reduction in vital capacity after light pre-medication with benzodiazepines. This effect is greater in patients with a body mass index exceeding 30 than in lean subjects, although this effect has not been shown to be statistically significant. Vital capacity reduction compared with baseline is significant in all subjects following surgery, and much more so in the obese as compared with overweight and non-obese patients. Vital capacity reduction is further compounded by site of surgery. Body cavity operations such as laparotomy result in a substantially greater reduction in vital capacity than body surface surgery, and this effect gets progressively greater with increasing body mass index. The combination of a body mass index greater than 30 kgm^{-2}, together with laparotomy, reduces vital capacity by more than 40% of baseline values. In lean subjects the reduction is only 10%.

3.4 **Cardiovascular changes**

The extent and severity of cardiovascular changes seen in obesity is highly variable. Important factors include both the body mass index and the duration of obesity, sometimes termed 'fat years'. The changes in cardiovascular physiology are complex and, as with so many features of pathophysiology in the obese, genetically determined. Consequently, there are many people who have accumulated numerous fat years, but who remain remarkably free of cardiovascular complications.

Common features include an increased blood volume compared with non-obese subjects, together with a raised cardiac output. As with the respiratory and metabolic changes, while the absolute values may be high, those corrected to body surface area are often normal or low. Morbidly obese patients (body mass index greater than 40) typically exhibit splanchnic blood flow 20% greater than that of lean individuals. Between 5 and 10% of subjects suffer severe hypertension, and up to 50% have moderate hypertension.

Animal work has shown that an increase in body mass index, whether genetic or experimentally induced, results in the increased myocardial fat content together with reduced contractility. When obesity is induced by dietary change, there is a complex pattern of myocardial gene expression which may in part explain the changes in adipocyte content and contractility. In obese animals, contractility is depressed both at baseline, and following beta-adrenergic stimulation, compared with non-obese animals. Both in animals and man, increasing body mass index and myocardial fat accumulation are also associated with endothelial dysfunction and increasing vascular resistance. These effects are thought to be mediated through a leptin-mediated increased expression of myocardial endothelin 1. There is a concomitant increase in oxygen stress and cardiac risk.

In man, myocardial fat correlates positively with waist-to-hip ratio and serum free fatty acid concentration. There is also positive association with left ventricular work. Epicardial fat content correlates positively with peripheral vascular resistance and negatively with myocardial contractility.

The reduction in contractility is not purely a mechanical effect due to the presence of adipocytes. Tissue culture work has shown that adipocytes are capable of exerting a profound effect on cardiac myocytes with an acute time course of action. The presence of adipocytes correlates with a reduction in fibre shortening as well as a reduction in peak intracellular calcium concentrations. This effect has been identified as being due to a humoral mediator of between 10 and 30 kPa.

Not all obese subjects, however, show functional myocardial impairments. Recent work in long-standing morbidly obese patients without myocardial complications has shown that there is also an increased left ventricular mass, this is appropriate to weight and sex. This patient group showed increased ejection fraction and mid systolic shortening compared with non-obese controls, suggesting a hyperdynamic state in systole.

3.5 The right heart

In addition to problems with the left ventricle and systemic vascular resistance, many obese patients develop right heart complications as a consequence of obstructive sleep apnoea and the obesity hypoventilation syndrome. Progressive elevation of pulmonary vascular resistance and pulmonary artery pressure results, eventually, in right ventricular overload and failure, with peripheral oedema and hepatic congestion. Right ventricular failure results in a reduced cardiac output and can progress rapidly to multiorgan failure. Consequently, it is important to seek out evidence of cor pulmonale or pulmonary hypertension during the pre-operative assessment.

In the most severely affected individuals, modest exercise (e.g., standing out of bed) or cardiovascular stress (intubation, surgery, post-operative pain) can induce cardiac decompensation. Sympathetic stimulation results in a rise in left ventricular end-diastolic pressure, myocardial ischaemia, elevated left atrial and pulmonary artery pressures, and right heart failure.

3.6 Gastrointestinal changes

There are numerous gastrointestinal changes associated with obesity. Many of these have pathological significance, and some are of immediate relevance in the perioperative period. Most important among these is the high prevalence of type 2 diabetes, which is often associated with severe insulin resistance and the metabolic syndrome.

There are specific intra-abdominal changes, particularly in those patients with an android fat distribution. There is an increase in intraperitoneal fat and in the bulk of the omentum. This results in increased intra-abdominal pressure, which is of significance both in terms of cardiorespiratory effects (reduced FRC, aorto-caval compression, etc.) and in terms of end organ effects. These include reduced tissue perfusion, and the potential for abdominal compartment syndrome following major surgery. This is often manifested as renal dysfunction in the bariatric surgery population.

There is involvement of the liver in the large majority of morbidly obese subjects coming to surgery. The prevalence of fatty liver is up to 90%. In addition to steatosis, a subset of patients develops inflammatory change and progress to steato hepatitis. The aetiology of this progression is unclear. There is a further group which progress to clinically significant cirrhosis. These changes have several practical implications. First of all, abdominal surgery may be rendered difficult by the physical enlargement of the liver, which in some cases extends into the contra-lateral iliac fossa. Steatosis also increases liver friability and the risk of haemorrhage. Coupled with this is the risk of portal hypertension and increased vascularity.

Hiatus hernia is common in morbid obesity. In one early series, 90% of patients studied had a gastric volume exceeding 25 mL at induction of anaesthesia, and a pH less than 2.5. By the criteria used in the obstetric anaesthesia, the majority of morbidly obese patients could be considered at risk of acid aspiration. Interestingly, this has seldom proved a problem in clinical practice. This may relate in part to differences in gastric motility between the pregnant and non-pregnant states.

Recent evidence suggests that morbidly obese patients may drink a significant volume of clear fluid (in one study, this amounted to 300 mL) up to 2 h before surgery, without any effect on gastric fluid volume or pH. These data suggest that traditional approaches to preoperative fasting may be too strict, and even counterproductive, in the morbidly obese population.

3.7 Conclusions

In summary, the physiology of obese patients varies considerably from that of non-obese individuals. These physiological changes seen in obesity encompass both obligate and variable features. Some of these give rise to specific pathologies and co-morbidities, which will be covered in later chapters. In many cases, they have a direct bearing on the conduct of anaesthesia and the ease and safety with which surgery can be performed. An understanding of the physiology of obesity is important to anaesthetise obese patients safely.

Further reading

Kankaanpaa M, Lehto HR, Parkka JP, *et al.* (2006). Myocardial triglyceride content and epicardial fat mass in human obesity: relationship to left ventricular function and serum free fatty acid levels. *J Clin Endocrinol Metab* **91**: 4689–95.

Lamounier-Zepter V, Ehrhart-Bornstein M, Karczewski P, Haase H, Bornstein SR, Morano I (2006). Human adipocytes attenuate cardio-myocyte contraction: characterization of an adipocyte-derived negative inotropic activity. *FASEB J.* **20**: 1653–9.

Pelosi P, Croci M, Ravagnan I, Tredici S, Pedoto A, Lissoni A, Gattinoni L (1998). The effects of body mass on lung volumes, respiratory mechanics, and gas exchange during general anesthesia. *Anesth Analg* **87**: 654–60.

Rusca M, Proietti S, Schnyder P, Frascarolo P, Hedenstierna G, Spahn DR, Magnusson L (2003). Prevention of Atelectasis formation during induction of general Anesthesia. *Anesth Analg* **97**: 1835–9.

von Ungern-Sternberg BS, Regli A, Schneider MC, Kunz F, Reber A (2004). Effect of obesity and site of surgery on perioperative lung volumes. *Br J Anaesth* **92**: 202–27.

Chapter 4

Obesity co-morbidities

> **Key points**
> - Not all obese patients suffer from co-morbidity.
> - In many cases, the presence of obesity-related co-morbidity is the reason a patient presents for surgery.
> - The majority of people with type 2 diabetes are overweight.
> - The waist circumference, rather than BMI, is the best predictor of type 2 diabetes.
> - Insulin therapy can be problematic in the morbidly obese.
> - There is a relationship between diet in the days prior to surgery and the degree of liver fatty infiltration at laparotomy.
> - In morbid obesity, moderate hypertension is present in 50% and severe hypertension in 10%.
> - There is a 14% additional chance of a cardiac event at 9-year follow-up for each BMI unit.
> - There is a BMI-related increase in the prevalence and severity of asthma.

Not all obese patients suffer from co-morbidity. However, the prevalence of obesity-related health problems increases with both the increasing body mass index (BMI) and the duration of obesity. Weight loss is generally helpful to control these conditions. In many situations, it may result in the complete resolution of co-morbidities. Nevertheless, conditions commonly thought of as being typical of obesity may also exist independently of obesity and so it is unreasonable to expect all such problems to resolve with weight loss.

In many cases, the presence of obesity-related co-morbidity is the reason for a patient to undergo surgery. For example, osteoarthritis is particularly common in obese subjects. This may affect the hip, the knee, or other joints. Obesity is thought to be the leading risk factor for osteoarthritis of the knee.

Many other co-morbidities may also either precipitate hospital treatment or result in complications during that treatment. Urinary incontinence, skin infections, oesophageal reflux, asthma, and other airway problems may either warrant treatment in their own right, or complicate anaesthesia and surgery for other conditions.

Much obesity-related co-morbidity is of particular interest in the perioperative period, either because they require specific intervention and management on the part of the anaesthetist, or because they modify perioperative and post-operative risk.

The most commonly encountered co-morbidities of immediate concern to the anaesthetist are diabetes and those affecting the respiratory and cardiovascular systems. Moderate or severe hypertension is frequently seen in the obese subjects. Other forms of cardiovascular disease, including coronary artery disease, also have an increased prevalence in this patient group. Likewise, problems such as airway obstruction, obstructive sleep apnoea, the obesity hypoventilation syndrome, and disorders of respiratory control frequently complicate long-standing morbid obesity, and especially patients who fall into the super obese and heavier categories.

Many co-morbidities interrelate with each other. For example, many individuals have gastric hyperacidity and an increased gastric residual volume. This, combined with sleep apnoea, snoring, and impaired upper airway reactivity, gives rise to nocturnal micro aspiration. This in turn precipitates lower airway reactivity and symptoms of asthma (Table 4.1).

4.1 **Diabetes**

The association between obesity and type 2 diabetes is well known. It has been confirmed in numerous studies, both cross-sectional and prospective. The majority of people with type 2 diabetes are overweight. Morbidly obese subjects, as compared with lean subjects, have an approximately 40 times greater risk of developing type 2 diabetes. The waist circumference, rather than BMI, is the best predictor of type 2 diabetes. This is probably because waist circumference correlates better with intra-abdominal fat, in itself an independent predictor of the metabolic syndrome. The metabolic syndrome is seen in many obese patients, and it is of immediate concern in the perioperative period. It consists of android type obesity, type 2 diabetes, often characterised by high blood sugars with insulin resistance, and an increased risk of cardiovascular disease. Women may additionally suffer polycystic ovaries, amenorrhoea, and hirsuitism.

Because of the problems of insulin resistance, multimodal therapy is often required to achieve adequate blood glucose control. Patients may describe their blood sugars as being 'controlled' by diet. This is seldom an accurate description of the situation.

Table 4.1 Commonly encountered obesity-related co-morbidity
Airway
Asthma
Obesity hypoventilation syndrome
Obstructive sleep apnoea
Pulmonary hypertension
Cardiovascular
Hypertension
Ischaemic heart disease
Cor pulmonale
Gastrointestinal and metabolic
Metabolic syndrome
Type 2 diabetes
Hyperlipidaemia
Acid reflux
Fatty liver
Steato-hepatitis
Musculo-skeletal
Osteoarthritis (hips and knees)
Compression fractures
Increased risk of injury
Other
Urinary incontinence
Skin infections
Candidiasis
Varicose veins
Lymphoedema
Poor self hygiene

Many others use oral hypoglycaemic drugs, often combining agents of different classes. Both sulphonylurea and biguanides are used. Typically, patients present with a drug history including compounds such as gliclazide taken in the morning, together with metformin taken at regular intervals throughout the day. In many cases a glita-zone has also been prescribed. Even those patients whose diabetic control has progressed to requiring insulin still frequently take met-formin. This is important to recognise, as it can contribute to an increased risk of lactic acidosis during and following surgery. Ideally, metformin should be discontinued at least 24 h prior to surgery. This often means that an insulin sliding scale regimen needs to be instituted.

Insulin therapy can be problematic in the morbidly obese. Because of insulin resistance, many subjects require very high doses of insulin and even that when such doses are administered, may still fail to gain adequate glucose control. The insulin administration route is important since subcutaneous drug absorption is frequently compromised. Carefully, intravenous insulin titration should be considered.

This is less of a problem when bariatric surgery is performed. Good glucose control is rapidly established following bariatric surgery, and more rapidly than could be expected as a consequence of weight loss. The reasons behind this are not clear.

Many morbidly obese patients suffer from a fatty liver. In the severe cases, this can progress to steato-hepatitis and eventually cirrhosis. It is not known why some patients suffer fatty infiltration without in entry consequences, while others develop an inflammatory condition. In addition to its general health consequences, a fatty liver is often problematic at laparotomy. First, this is because of the increased size of the liver, which can obstruct access to other intra-abdominal organs. Second, the tissues can be extremely friable, with a risk of liver rupture and major intra-operative haemorrhage.

There is a relationship between diet in the days prior to surgery and the degree of fatty infiltration in the liver. A low carbohydrate, protein-rich diet for even a short period of time can have a dramatic effect on reducing the bulk and fat content of the liver. There is also a relationship between the use of oral hypoglycaemic drugs and hepatic steatosis. Drugs such as metformin appear to exacerbate the problem, while agents such as rosiglitazone ameliorate it.

4.2 **Hypertension**

There is a positive correlation between blood pressure and increasing BMI. The 2003 Health Survey for England suggested that the increase in systolic blood pressure with obesity is around 6 mmHg. It has been estimated that moderate hypertension is present in 50% of patients with morbid obesity, and severe hypertension in 5–10% of such individuals. There are also racial differences in susceptibility to obesity-related hypertension; after correction for age and gender, there is a greater prevalence of hypertension among black people than whites for each BMI interval.

However, it is not clear that obesity *per se* is a cause of hypertension. Although weight gain is associated with an increased risk of developing hypertension, 'weight cycling', in which weight is alternately and repeatedly gained and lost, is not associated with the development of hypertension. Conceivably, obesity merely alters the time course of hypertension. Data taken from the Swedish Obese Subjects (SOS) study suggested that, while weight loss was followed by resolution of hypertension, this improvement in blood pressure was not permanent in all subjects. It lasted around 10 years, before the blood pressure in previously hypertensive individuals rose again to hypertensive values.

Weight loss is associated with a reduction in the number of drugs needed to control blood pressure.

In the perioperative period, there is relatively little evidence that moderate hypertension is associated with increased perioperative morbidity or mortality. However, it is associated with increased blood pressure lability during surgery. This can be a significant issue during anaesthesia for the morbidly obese. Many patients are difficult to intubate, and the prolonged stress of laryngoscopy may lead to blood pressure surge. Following this, there may be a precipitate fall in blood pressure, either associated with the supine position and aortocaval compression, or associated with the use of reverse Trendelenberg position (often employed to aid ventilation and to improve functional residual capacity). Those whose hypertension is adequately treated, and who are appropriately volume resuscitated, are less susceptible to swings in blood pressure.

4.3 **Ischaemic heart disease**

There is an increasing prevalence of ischaemic heart disease with rising BMI. A recent Korean study quantified this, after multivariate adjustment, as a 14% additional chance of a cardiac event at 9 year follow-up for each BMI unit. In asymptomatic French middle-aged men, larger abdominal girth (but not BMI) was associated with increased risk of sudden death, independent of known cardiovascular risk factors.

This is clearly of concern to the anaesthetist. Moreover, because of a sedentary lifestyle, there is not always a clear history of angina or other symptoms. Chest pain, when present, may be confused with reflux. Likewise, smote angina presenting as breathlessness years of fun easily confused with the effects of being overweight or suffering obesity-related asthma. Resting echocardiography and ECG often fail to diagnose underlying ischaemic heart disease. To compound this, exercise testing is frequently impracticable.

There is an increased prevalence of risk factors for coronary heart disease with increasing obesity. These include diabetes and hypertension (see above) as well as alterations in lipid profile. Smoking may also carry a greater risk in the obese than in lean individuals.

Some recent studies have claimed that, in patients with ischaemic heart disease, there is a reduced perioperative risk when beta-blockers are introduced in the perioperative period. These data do not relate specifically to obese subjects, in whom specific studies have not yet been carried out.

4.4 **Lipids**

Obesity is linked with higher serum cholesterol concentrations, as well as an unfavourably low ratio of high-density lipoprotein to low-density lipoprotein. As with many other obesity-related risk factors, this tendency is worse in those with central and obesity (the android fat distribution pattern) as compared to those with a gynaecoid fat distribution pattern. This is one of the reasons why patients with an android fat distribution are at greater risk of coronary heart disease. The lipid abnormality becomes more severe with increasing BMI. It has been suggested that reduction in low-density lipoprotein concentrations achieved by therapy with statins is equivalent to that of a 40 kg reduction in weight. Although both approaches may be desirable, the scope for weight loss in the period between listing for surgery and carrying out an elective operation is strictly limited.

A consequence of this is that an increasing number of patients presenting for anaesthesia and surgery are taking statins. Statins may have important effects other than modifying lipid profiles. These include both beneficial effects, such as reduction in the pro-inflammatory response, and potentially harmful effects, such as the derangement of liver function tests, and, very rarely, drug-induced hepatitis. It has been suggested that acute discontinuation of statins in the perioperative period may be harmful. Firm evidence for this yet to emerge, although the idea seems both logical and attractive. Therefore, the reasonable and cautious approach seems to be to continue statins except in those patients with deranged liver function tests. Many morbidly obese patients suffer acute fatty liver, and therefore may be at greater risk than the non-obese population.

4.5 **Smoking**

In general, all patients presenting for anaesthesia and surgery should be discouraged from smoking, at least in the perioperative period. The risks associated with smoking are multiple and compound than those of obesity. Where possible, obese patients presenting for elective surgery should be offered help with smoking cessation for several weeks prior to surgery.

The risks to which they are included those relating specifically to the lungs and airway, those relating to the carriage and delivery of oxygen to the tissues, and those relating to cardiovascular risk.

Smokers are at increased risk of retention of secretions due to reduced ciliary motility. It is usually necessary to stop smoking for several weeks for ciliary motility to be regained. This is particularly important in overweight patients. The typical 'early morning smoker's cough' suffered by many is related to an overnight accumulation of secretions, together with a partial recovery of ciliary activity and airway reflexes. Many smokers deal with this early morning cough by smoking a cigarette. This results in suppression of airway reflexes again, and a reduction in the tendency to cough. It also results in increased retention of sputum and secretions. Both heightened airway reactivity and secretion retention are undesirable in the perioperative period; hence, the desirability of smoking cessation for at least two weeks prior to anaesthesia.

In addition to the effects on airway reflexes and reactivity, secretion retention can result in reduced functional residual capacity. There is also reduced functional residual capacity with increasing BMI. This situation is further compounded by anaesthesia and the supine position. Both smoking and obesity increase the alveolar to arterial oxygen tension gradient. The combination of the two is clearly undesirable.

Smokers have increased carboxy haemoglobin levels. This, combined with increased blood viscosity, reduces delivery of oxygen to the tissues. Reduced tissue oxygen tension in obesity surgery is associated with an increased complication rate. Stopping smoking even for a few days can help to reduce carboxy haemoglobin levels. It is likely that this is linked with a concomitant reduction in perioperative risk.

Many obese patients, when advised to stop smoking, suggest that this may be unwise. They point out, correctly, that when they have given up smoking in the past, they have gained weight. There is good evidence to support this observation. However, the effects on metabolism and risk are not quite as simple. Data from several countries suggest that those who smoke, while they lose weight, also suffer an unfavourable increase in the waist-to-hip ratio (in other words, an increase in central as opposed to peripheral obesity). People who have never smoked have the most favourable waist-to-hips ratios, ex-smokers performing less well, and current smokers faring worst of all. So, in terms of risk modification, how important is it for obese patients to stop smoking? In terms of perioperative risk, the issues are quite clear. However, in terms of overall health improvement, data from the United States suggest that obesity itself has a much greater effect on the risk of chronic health conditions such as ischaemic heart disease than does smoking.

4.6 **Asthma**

There is an increased incidence of episodes of asthma attacks in obese subjects. Furthermore, there also seems to be an increase in the prevalence of background wheezing and chronic asthma. In adults of both genders, there is a BMI-related increase in both the prevalence and severity of asthma. This is also seen in children, where in a recent Spanish study of 20,000 children aged 6 and 7, there was an increased odds ratio for asthma of 2.35 in obese girls. Interestingly, while diet was an important factor in boys, obesity did not seem to increase the risk of asthma.

The reasons behind this are thought to be multiple; factors such as sleep apnoea and partial airway obstruction seemed to play a role. It seems likely that acid reflux and micro aspiration resulting in airway injury are also important. Other factors include peripheral airway closure, particularly in the tidal volume of breathing. This is thought to result in increased sheer stresses in the airway with a resulting pro-inflammatory response. Several recently published series suggest that bariatric surgery results in between 80 and 100% resolution of symptoms in patients with obesity-related asthma. Perioperative management includes appropriate investigation, and consideration for the use of anti-reflux and antacid therapies, and strategies to maintain an 'open lung'. These could include treatment of sleep apnoea with continuous positive airway pressure in the preoperative period, anti-inflammatory and bronchodilator therapies.

4.7 **Conclusions**

Obese patients presenting for anaesthesia and surgery are likely to suffer a number of obesity-related co-morbidities. The majority of these are related not only to the severity of overweight or obesity, but also to their duration. Most require independent consideration and management in the perioperative period. The effects of these co-morbidities may be more severe and less predictable than in non-obese individuals. Appropriate investigation and control of obesity-related conditions are best handled by a multidisciplinary team approach.

Further reading

Beuther DA, Sutherland ER. (2007). Overweight, obesity and incident asthma: a meta-analysis of prospective epidemiologic studies. *Am J Respir Crit Care Med* **18**: [Epub ahead of print].

Garcia-Marcos L, Miner Canflanca I, Batlles Garrido J, *et al.* (2007). The relationship of asthma and rhinoconjunctivitis with obesity, exercise and Mediterranean diet in Spanish schoolchildren 6–7 years old. *Thorax* Jan 24; [Epub ahead of print].

Peluso L, Vanek VW (2007). Efficacy of gastric bypass in the treatment of obesity-related comorbidities. *Nutr Clin Pract* **22**: 22–8.

Sjostrom CD, Peltonen M, Wedel H, Sjostrom L (2000). Differentiated long-term effects of intentional weight loss on diabetes and hypertension. *Hypertension* **36**: 20–5.

Torgerson JS, Sjostrom L (2001). The Swedish Obese Subjects (SOS) study – rationale and results. *Int J Obes Relat Metab Disord* **25** Suppl 1: S2–S4.

Wild SH, Byrne CD (2006). Risk factors for diabetes and coronary heart disease. ABC of obesity. *Br Med J* **333**: 1009–11.

Woolf AD, Breedveld F, Kvien TK (2006). Controlling the obesity epidemic is important for maintaining musculoskeletal health. *Ann Rheum Dis* **65**: 1401–2.

Chapter 5

Disorders of sleep and respiratory control in obesity: perioperative assessment and management

Many obese patients suffer from disorders of respiratory control. These are divided into two main categories: the obesity hypoventilation syndrome and obstructive sleep apnoea. Patients may suffer from both conditions simultaneously. Both conditions have major implications for all the perioperative management of obese and overweight patients.

5.1 **The obesity hypoventilation syndrome**

In the obesity hypoventilation syndrome, there is altered respiratory control in the awake state. The syndrome is defined as an elevated arterial carbon dioxide tension while awake, in association with a body mass index above 30 kgm^{-2}. Most definitions specify a partial pressure of carbon dioxide greater than 6 kPa or 45 mmHg. The obesity hypoventilation syndrome can only be diagnosed in the absence of other causes of elevated carbon dioxide tension (Table 5.1).

Table 5.1 **Diagnostic criteria for the obesity hypoventilation syndrome**

Diagnosis of obesity hypoventilation syndrome
• Absence of other causes of hypercarbia
• Body mass index greater than 30 kgm^{-2}
• Awake arterial pCO$_2$ > 6 kPa (45 mmHg)
• Obstructive sleep apnoea (present in 85% of cases)

It is important to measure carbon dioxide partial pressure when the patient is awake, so that individuals with nocturnal hypoventilation or the obesity-related sleep apnoea syndrome can be adequately excluded.

Obesity hypoventilation syndrome is common, and its prevalence rises with increasing body mass index. It has been estimated that, in an American population, the prevalence is as high as 31% in subjects with a body mass index above 35 kgm^{-2}. The precise aetiology and underlying pathological factors are unclear. However, it has been postulated that there may be a causal relationship between leptin insensitivity and the obesity hypoventilation syndrome mediated via a hypothalamic pathway. These data are largely supported by animal work in which mice with diet-induced obesity develop an increased respiratory drive associated with increased leptin levels, whereas leptin-deficient mice fail to do so. There are some limited human data correlating leptin levels with respiratory drive.

The obesity hypoventilation syndrome is often a 'missed diagnosis'. Many patients presenting for surgery suffer from this syndrome, and are at increased risk of perioperative respiratory depression. Arterial blood gases awake may confirm the diagnosis. In other patients, it may be possible to estimate the arterial carbon dioxide tension from the awake end tidal carbon dioxide percentage in the expired gas. The frequency with which this returns to a value above 6 kPa is surprising. The response of the diaphragm electromyogram to an increasing arterial concentration of carbon dioxide is used as a measure of central respiratory drive (ΔEMG/ΔpCO$_2$). In simple obesity, there is an increased diaphragmatic response; whereas in patients with the obesity hypoventilation syndrome, the diaphragm electromyogram response to changes in carbon dioxide concentration resembles that of nonobese individuals. These findings are consistent with the view that obese subjects, because of the mechanical restriction to respiration, develop an increased respiratory drive. Those who fail to do so become hypercarbic.

Several case series have confirmed an increased morbidity and even mortality resulting from the obesity hypoventilation syndrome. There is an increased prevalence of pulmonary hypertension and right heart failure. Several series have confirmed increased in-hospital mortality in patients with the obesity hypoventilation syndrome admitted for other reasons. In the majority of cases, those who died succumbed as a result either of progressive respiratory failure or pulmonary embolism.

Currently, there is no effective treatment for the obesity hypoventilation syndrome other than weight loss. Progesterone has been suggested as a therapy, as it is demonstrated to increase central carbon dioxide sensitivity. However, there are no data to confirm sustained symptomatic improvement or better long-term outcomes. Consequently, progesterone is not currently a recommended therapy for the obesity hypoventilation syndrome.

5.2 **Obstructive sleep apnoea**

Obstructive sleep apnoea is very common in obese subjects. Implications for the anaesthetist fall into the usual categories of pre-operative, perioperative, and post-operative. The diagnosis is generally suspected on the basis of history. In addition to this, a number of special investigations can be performed to quantify more certainly both its presence and its severity. These investigations can best be performed in a properly equipped sleep studies laboratory. There are alternative, simpler devices used in clinical practice for quantifying sleep disorders and hypoxia, although these are somewhat less reliable than a formal sleep laboratory assessment.

The syndrome is characterised by intermittent periods of airway obstruction, tidal volume reduction, and breathing cessation during deep sleep. These may result in hypoxia, often with severe arterial desaturation. Episodes are usually terminated by sudden arousal or awakening, which results in the disruption of sleep, and especially of deep slow wave (SWS or Non-REM) and rapid eye movement (REM) sleep. This is significant, as it often results in daytime somnolence.

Obstructive sleep apnoea syndrome is defined by the apnoea-hypopnoea index. This is the number of episodes of apnoea or significant hypopnoea per hour of sleep. A count of five or above defines the syndrome, and is associated with increasing daytime sleepiness. In the most severe cases, the apnoea-hypopnoea index can exceed 100.

In adults, obstructive sleep apnoea has a roughly 4-fold greater prevalence in men than in women, and a 4-fold greater prevalence in those with a body mass index above 30 kgm^{-2}. The average age at presentation is around 50 years. Up to 90% of cases are undiagnosed. Data from North America suggest that 24% of men and 9% of women have an apnoea-hypopnoea index greater than 5, and 16% of men and 22% of women suffer daytime hypersomnolence. Sleep apnoea is also seen in children, in whom it is associated with obesity or adeno-tonsilar hypertrophy.

Retrospective and cross-sectional studies have demonstrated a clear association between the obstructive sleep apnoea and cardiovascular morbidity. However, most of these have not confirmed a causal relationship. Indeed, because of the presence of other cardiovascular risk factors in this patient population, it is likely that obstructive sleep apnoea is not itself the cause. The possible exception to this is arterial hypertension. The apnoea-hypopnoea index alone is a poor guide to the need for clinical intervention, as it correlates poorly with symptomatology and co-morbidity.

Patients generally present with a characteristic history. Most cannot remember sleeping poorly, or waking up at night, although they may describe increased nocturnal frequency of micturition independent of prostatic symptoms. There is generally a history of loud snoring. This history is often volunteered not by the patient but by their partner. In many cases, the snoring is sufficiently loud to prevent the patient's partner from sleeping, often resulting in the partner spending the night in a different room. Typically, there is a repeating pattern through the night of increasing crescendo snoring, followed by silence with paradoxical respiratory motion. Recovery is accompanied by coughing, choking, and sometimes by sudden awakening. The patient's partner may also describe how the patient 'stops breathing' and then suddenly wakes up. Sometimes, the partner describes having to shake and awaken the patient to prompt recommencement of breathing. Episodes may be accompanied by restlessness and gross movement of the limbs. Generally, the patient has little or no recollection of these episodes.

The patient may describe waking in the morning with a headache, after an apparently good night's sleep. Most subjects describe mood and affect disturbances, an inability to concentrate, aggression, and a decline in decision-making skills. The patient may also relate feeling tired and sleepy during the day. In severe cases, this results in the subject falling asleep whenever sitting to perform a task. Examples of this include falling asleep at their desks, falling asleep while watching television, and falling asleep while driving. Indeed, patients who suffer obstructive sleep apnoea are estimated to be involved in a between 3 and 20 times as many motor accidents as patients without sleep apnoea. The road death rate attributable to obstructive sleep apnoea is said to exceed that due to alcohol.

A number of factors contribute to obstructive sleep apnoea in the obese. These include narrowing of the airway and palatal area, together with fat infiltration between the airway and constrictor muscles. Magnetic resonance scans of the airway in patients with obstructive sleep apnoea characteristically show white 'flashes' of fats between the medial and lateral pterygoids. There may also be anatomical disorders or an abnormal position of the mandible. Consequently, there are multiple abnormalities simultaneously which results in reduction of airway calibre, and increased compliance (reduced 'stiffness') of the wall of the oro-pharynx. During the inspiration, there is narrowing and collapse of the airway despite appropriate upper airway muscular tone. A subatmospheric pressure is generated in the airway, giving rise to atelectasis and collapse in the respiratory tree.

Over time, the obstructive sleep apnoea syndrome results in a 'pathological triad' of increased inspiratory effort, reduced oxygenation, and hypercarbia. Increased inspiratory effort is a potential cause of reflux and aspiration, resulting in increased lower airway reactivity and asthma. Reduced oxygenation can result in hypoxic pulmonary vasoconstriction, and ultimately pulmonary hypertension and cor pulmonale. Systemic hypertension, and arguably, other cardiovascular side effects, may also complicate chronic nocturnal hypoxia. Chronic hypoxia can also blunt the ventilatory response to hypoxia, resulting in reduced respiratory drive both asleep and awake. This is of particular significance in the immediate post-operative period.

A chronically elevated nocturnal carbon dioxide tension can blunt the response to hypercarbia and result in reduced pulmonary compliance. As with chronic hypoxia, the implications for surgery and anaesthesia are extremely important in the more severely affected individual.

Children with obstructive sleep apnoea usually have a history of daytime attention deficit and hyperactivity, coupled with nocturnal restlessness, night sweats, and enuresis. The parents usually described how their child sleeps poorly and restlessly. The child breathes through the mouth, with the head and neck hyperextended. There may be paradoxical breathing: with inspiration, there is a seesaw motion of the abdomen, and rib recession in younger children.

5.3 Investigation of obstructive sleep apnoea

Investigation of obstructive sleep apnoea can be divided into out-patient and inpatient categories. Preliminary assessment is performed in the outpatient setting. This includes a detailed history together with the use of questionnaires (such as the Epworth sleepiness scale). This can be followed by a home oximetry and accompanied by neck measurement. Some centres also employed lateral cephalometry.

These measures are followed, where indicated, by formal inpatient assessment. Generally, this comprises polysomnography. Home oximetry, even when coupled with other simple tests of respiratory function while sleeping (e.g., nasal flow measurements) has a poor predictive value. It is highly sensitive for obstructive sleep apnoea (in one study, 98%), but has a low specificity (48%). The performance of simple outpatient measurements can be improved substantially by combining them with a risk index. The clinical probability of a positive test for sleep apnoea is substantially lower in people whose adjusted neck circumference is less than 43 cm. Patients with a neck circumference between 43 and 48 cm have a moderate probability of a positive test for sleep apnoea, and those with a neck circumference above 48 cm, a high probability. The adjusted neck circumference is made up of the measured circumference in centimetres, to which 4 cm is added if the patient is hypertensive, and 3 cm is added for habitual snoring, or for those who are reported to suffer 'choking' most nights.

Polysomnography is the technique of choice for investigating moderate and high-risk patients. The device records many features of sleep. The stage and depth of sleep are determined by electroencephalography, electrooculography (to define periods of REM sleep), and the electromyogram. Simultaneously, oxygen saturation and airflow are recorded. Some systems additionally record abdominal paradoxical movement, limb movement, and postural shift. Different systems use their own methods for measuring breathing. The precise criteria for defining respiratory disturbance (including hypopnoea) are not standardised.

A typical tracing recorded during obstructive sleep apnoea shows chaotic behaviour, with repeated episodes of arterial desaturation (of varying severity) accompanied by significant pulse rate variability. Episodes of awakening are accompanied by a return of arterial oxygen saturation towards normal values (Figure 5.1).

5.4 **Treatment of obstructive sleep apnoea**

Where patients are due to present for elective surgery, pre-operative treatment of obstructive sleep apnoea is a feasible option and may significantly reduce such physiological derangements as reduced oxygen and carbon dioxide sensitivity, and right heart failure. By facilitating a return to normal sleep patterns, with a normal

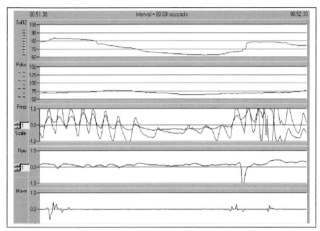

Figure 5.1 Polysomnography data showing arterial oxygen saturation, respiratory rate, airflow, and movement during an episode of apnoea. Courtesy of Professor Chris Dodds, Clinical Director, South Tees NHS Trust Sleep Laboratory.

proportion of nocturnal REM sleep, there is theoretically a reduced risk of opioid-induced respiratory depression in the post-operative period. Clearly, elective treatment of obstructive sleep apnoea for patients presenting for surgery is only possible in the elective situation. Nevertheless, it is feasible to introduce some treatment modalities, for example, continuous positive airway pressure (CPAP), in the immediate perioperative period.

Treatment of obstructive sleep apnoea is only that it does not represent a 'cure'. A number of treatment options have been tried. Foremost among these is the use of CPAP. Polysomnography before and after treatment with CPAP showed that it brings about an immediate reversal of airway obstruction, apnoea, and hypopnoea. It also reduces daytime symptoms and results in improvements in quality-of-life. CPAP therapy is reasonably well tolerated, with short-term compliance reaching 80%. However, not all patients find this suitable as a long-term treatment. Many suffer symptoms such as nasal congestion. Others find that the device is uncomfortable or noisy, and keeps them awake at night. Those patients who tolerate CPAP the best are those whose sleep patterns are worst before institution of therapy. This group of patients report dramatic improvements in the quality-of-life.

Other specific treatments include the use of oral appliances and devices to advance the mandible. Prostheses can also be fitted to the teeth or dental arches which can either reposition the mandible, or modify the shape of the retro palatal airway. Such devices are more effective than placebo, but do not outperform CPAP.

Airway surgery is also an option in a small minority of patients. Procedures such as palato-uvuloplasty and hemiglossectomy have been performed. According to the Cochrane reviewers, there are insufficient trials to support these procedures over the use of airway prostheses or CPAP.

Conservative treatment, including weight loss, is probably the most effective strategy after CPAP. Avoiding sleeping in the supine position, avoiding alcohol prior to sleeping, and avoiding sedative medication have all been shown to improve obstructive sleep apnoea. A 10% reduction in weight is associated with a 26% reduction in the apnoea-hyponoea index in the observational data. In one series, bariatric surgery was associated with a reduction in the mean apnoea-hypopnoea index from 97 to 11. It is not clear whether these improvements are sustained. Some authors have reported a partial rebound in the apnoea-hypopnoea index, despite patients maintaining a lower weight.

5.5 **Conclusions**

Both obstructive sleep apnoea and the obesity hypoventilation syndrome result in physiological derangements that increase perioperative risk. Most importantly, they contribute to altered hypoxic drive and reduced sensitivity to hypercarbia. These have the potential to increase the risk of perioperative hypoxia and in extreme cases may give rise to respiratory arrest. Where patients present for elective surgery, the risk attributable to obstructive sleep apnoea can be partially mitigated by the introduction of CPAP in the weeks leading up to surgery. In the case of emergency surgery, CPAP may still be of value in the immediate perioperative period.

Further reading

Flemons WW (2002). Sleep apnea. *NEJM* **347**(7): 498–504.

Olson AL, Zwillich C (2005). The obesity hypoventilation syndrome. *Am J Med* **118**(9): 948–56.

Poulain M, Doucet M, Major GC, Drapeau V, Series F, Boulet LP, Tremblay A, Maltais F (2006). The effect of obesity on chronic respiratory diseases: pathophysiology and therapeutic strategies. *CMAJ* **174**(9): 1293–9.

Scheuller M, Weider D (2001). Bariatric surgery for treatment of sleep apnea syndrome in 15 morbidly obese patients: long-term results. *Otolaryngol Head Neck Surg* **125**(4): 299–302.

Chapter 6

Anaesthetic pharmacology and obesity

> **Key points**
> - Many drugs behave differently in obese and non-obese subjects.
> - This results from both pharmacokinetic and pharmacodynamic factors.
> - mg/kg doses provided by manufacturers are based on total body weight in the lean patient population and have limited relevance to total body weight in the obese.
> - Drug dose may be based on total body weight, ideal body weight, or lean body mass depending on the drug.
> - There is great variability between individual subjects.

Many drugs behave differently in obese and non-obese subjects. The reasons for this are multiple and complex. They encompass both pharmacokinetic and pharmacodynamic factors. These in turn inter-relate both with patient pathophysiology and drug physico-chemical properties. This means that, in obesity, the activity profile of many agents cannot easily be predicted. Moreover, most studies in the literature relating to drug action in obesity are based on small sample sizes or animal work, and there is a remarkable degree of inconsistency between them. The situation is not helped by the data provided by drug companies. Manufacturers' data sheets are limited by the fact that they are part of the licensing process for the drug, and therefore reflect data derived from large clinical trials in 'normal' subjects. Manufacturers are not at liberty to include details of small clinical trials, which have not been submitted to the licensing authorities in support of the original application for a product licence.

6.1 Pharmacodynamic considerations

Theoretically, there may be significant pharmacodynamic changes in the obese. This is due to changes in receptor populations and activity either as a cause or as a consequence of obesity. Altered receptor expression and function are seen together with changes in concentrations of endogenous ligands, in the central nervous system as well as in the periphery. Some of these pharmacological changes have been discussed in Chapter 2.

Although a number of interesting and potentially significant changes in receptor populations and function have been described, their practical implications for pharmacological manipulation have been explored only in so far as they relate to the treatment of obesity. They have not been extensively studied in terms of their implications for anaesthesia.

Receptor populations, which behave differently in obesity, include opioid receptors, GABA receptors, and the peripheral sympathetic nervous system, in particular, the beta adrenoreceptor. All of these have interesting and potentially significant implications for the behaviour of drugs used in anaesthesia and critical care. However, clinical data are lacking.

6.2 **Pharmacokinetic considerations**

Drug doses may require modification in the obese subject owing to changes in the key pharmacokinetic variables. In general, drug absorption in the obesity, whether by the oral intravenous route, is very similar to that in non-obese subjects. Absorption by the intra-muscular and subcutaneous routes is less reliable in obese subjects than in lean individuals, because of relatively poor tissue blood flow, particularly to the peripheries.

There are however important differences both in volume of distri-bution and clearance of drugs in the obese. These, in turn, result in complex changes in effect site concentration, terminal half-life, and context-sensitive half-time according to the interaction between variables. There is great variability not only between drugs with different dissociation constants, lipid solubility, and protein-binding characteristics, but also between individual patients, even those with similar body mass indices and fat distribution. These effects may be further obscured by drug-drug interactions.

Package inserts and other prescribing data in standard texts and pharmacopoeias generally relate dosage to body weight, or in some cases to body surface area. However, these data are based on patients whose weight lies close to the population mean. Although this may be appropriate for some drugs in morbidly obese patients, it is not clearly applicable to all pharmacologically active compounds. There has been considerable debate in the literature about appropriate adjustment of the 'weight' value employed for this purpose.

6.3 **What body weight should be used?**

The most appropriate body weight value differs according to physicochemical properties of the drug as well as specific pharmacokinetic considerations in the patient. A number of general principles underline this. Many drugs have an altered volume of distribution in obesity. In principle, lipid-soluble drugs are likely to have a substantially increased volume of distribution, in proportion to the increased proportion of body fat. Likewise, highly water-soluble drugs are likely to display a lesser difference in volume of distribution between obese and non-obese subjects.

Those drugs, which are highly protein bound, may also show greater similarities between obese and non-obese individuals. Differences in protein binding can account for complex changes in the volume of distribution. Albumin binding is similar between obese and lean individuals. However, volume of distribution is influenced by the presence of other plasma proteins including alpha-1 acid glycoprotein, by fatty acids, and by triglycerides. Because these are increased in obesity, acidic drugs tend to have a similar free fraction in both obese and non-obese subjects, whereas basic drugs have an increased free fraction.

'Ideal body weight' is a function of a subject's gender and height. For some drugs, the ideal body weight may be appropriate to use when calculating a dosing schedule. This might seem appealing in the case of a drug of low-fat solubility, which would not be expected to distribute into the adipose tissue compartment. In practice, however, this rule frequently does not apply when tested clinically.

The situation is more complicated when considering drugs with moderate lipid solubility. Simplistically, their volume of distribution might be expected to increase with increasing weight. This would suggest that volume of distribution, and hence dosing, should be related to total body weight. This view, however, is an oversimplification. There is an old song which says that 'man is made of muscle and blood and skin and bone'. Obese subjects have increased adipose tissue content, but this is not simply fat mass *added to* the ideal body weight. There is also an increase in the mass of other body constituents and tissue compartments ('muscle and blood and skin', etc.). This means that the mass of the non-adipose tissue compartments cannot adequately be described by the ideal body weight. The size of these components is somewhat greater than ideal body weight in the obese, and is described as the 'lean body mass'.

Whether the ideal body weight, lean body mass, or total body weight is used in drug dose calculations depends on the compartmental kinetics of the drug in question, as the dose adjustment from the recommended 'milligrams per kilogram' regimen depends on the relative size of the compartments in obese patients, together with the relevance of each compartment for any given drug. Because of the variability between studies, and the difficulty in deciding which 'body weight' to use, several investigators have related drug dose to 'corrected body weight'. The corrected body weight is a clinical 'rough and ready' estimation, but is not evidence based. It is calculated by adding 40% of the excess weight to the ideal body weight.

A number of nomograms have been published which describe the relationship between total body weight, ideal body weight, and lean body mass for men and women of different body weights. None of these is entirely satisfactory, as they fail to take account of differences in fat distribution. Several simple formulae for calculating relative weights are commonly used in clinical practice. These are summarised in Table 6.1.

Table 6.1 Definitions of modified body weights used for dose calculations
IBW (kg) = height (cm) − x
(where x = 100 for adult males and 105 for adult females)
LBM = $1.1x$ (weight) − 128 (weight/height)^2 ....(Male)
LBM = $1.07x$ (weight) − 148 (weight/height)^2 ....(Female)
IBW: ideal body weight; LBM: lean body mass.

6.4 Drug elimination and clearance

There is a relationship between increasing obesity and increasing cardiac output. Because of the obesity hypoventilation syndrome there may be a relative (but not absolute) reduction in the alveolar minute volume as compared with non-obese subjects. Together, these factors mean that both uptake and elimination of drugs by the inhalational route take a longer time to achieve steady-state concentration than is the case in non-obese individuals. Coupled with this, there is increased organ blood flow to key organs involved in drug disposition and elimination.

Compared with lean individuals, obese subjects have an increased absolute renal blood flow and glomerular filtration rate. This results in increased renal clearance of many compounds in absolute terms. However, the relationship between this and elimination half-life depends on factors such as changes in the volume of distribution, which may be highly complex.

Likewise, there may be in absolute terms a substantially increased splanchnic blood flow, and consequently increased hepatic blood flow. This may result in absolute increased delivery of drug to the liver. The effect on drug metabolism is further modified by structural and functional changes in the liver seen in obesity. Many obese individuals suffer fatty infiltration of the liver; in severe cases, this can progress to non-alcoholic steato hepatitis and in some cases fibrosis and cirrhosis. Ultimately, these changes can result in altered hepatic synthetic function (with consequent changes in plasma proteins and volumes of drug distribution) and reduced drug metabolism.

Long before these changes occur, there are functional changes in hepatic drug handling attributable to obesity. Despite fatty infiltration of the liver, there is little measurable change in phase 1 metabolism (redox reactions). This means that the inactivation of active compounds by the liver is similar between obese and non-obese individuals. Obesity and fatty infiltration of the liver are associated with an increase in phase 2 metabolism for many compounds (conjugation reactions). Both active and inactive compounds are converted more rapidly to water-soluble forms; hence, their terminal half-life is accelerated.

6.5 Inhalational anaesthetic agents

Theoretically, for all inhalational agents, there may be a prolonged time to achieving steady state in obese as compared with non-obese subjects, because of an increased cardiac output to minute volume ratio. The pharmacokinetics of inhalational anaesthetic agents can be predicted according to their blood–gas partition coefficient and oil–gas (i.e., lipid) solubility coefficient. Consequently, there are differences in both uptake and elimination between lean and obese subjects, which are specific to individual inhalational agents. In all patients, whether lean or obese, agents with a low blood gas solubility coefficient will approach steady state (during both uptake and elimination) more rapidly than agents with a high blood gas solubility coefficient. This means that, in obese patients in whom a rapid postoperative recovery is desirable, agents with lower blood gas solubility represent a more attractive option than those with high blood gas solubility. This might favour, for example, agents such as desflurane, nitrous oxide, and sevoflurane over those such as halothane or ether.

The time to achieve a clinically appropriate effect-site concentration for volatile anaesthetic agents is a function primarily of the blood gas solubility coefficient. This is because equilibration between the lung, blood, and brain compartments is relatively rapid. Effect site pseudo steady-state concentration is rapidly achieved.

During the elimination phase, however, lipid solubility (and hence the oil–gas partition coefficient) plays a greater role. In the obese subject, because there is a larger fat component, the absolute mass of inhalational agent distributed to this compartment is greater than in the non-obese subject. Agents with higher lipid solubility achieve higher fat component concentrations. Consequently, for such agents, there is a greater absolute mass of drug at steady state in the obese than in the non-obese subject. Consequently, the elimination half-time is prolonged. In practice, because blood flow to adipose tissue compartments is relatively small, the rate at which lipid-soluble volatile agents are redistributed to these compartments is correspondingly low. This means that steady state is only achieved in adipose compartments, in the case of highly lipid-soluble inhalational agents, after a prolonged anaesthetic (mostly exceeding the clinical time range).

An interesting consequence of this is that lipid-soluble volatile agents show a longer recovery time in obese than in non-obese subjects, and this difference is further accentuated according to the duration of anaesthesia. It is interesting to consider the theoretical differences between an agent such as desflurane (low blood solubility, low lipid solubility) and cyclopropane (low blood solubility, high lipid solubility). The latter would be expected to give rapid induction and recovery from anaesthesia in lean subjects, a similar profile of induction but slower recovery in obese subjects, and a very prolonged recovery after a prolonged anaesthetic in an obese subject. In contrast, desflurane behaves similarly in subjects of different body habitus and after different durations of anaesthesia.

The very favourable induction and recovery characteristics of desflurane (and, to a lesser extent, sevoflurane) have lead clinicians to propose that these are the inhalational agents of choice for use in the obese. However, despite their attractiveness in clinical practice, there are theoretical concerns, which may limit their desirability. These relate to the increased generation of their major metabolites (including inorganic fluoride) in obese individuals as compared with lean subjects. These objections are probably largely theoretical, as only one case of desflurane hepatotoxicity has been reported. This is in strong contrast to the older agents, and in particular halothane and enflurane, both of which are associated with clinically important generation of metabolites in the obese. In the case of halothane, this leads to a clinically important increased risk of hepatic dysfunction, and in the case of enflurane a theoretical risk of renal failure. Isoflurane has slightly less favourable induction and recovery characteristics than the desflurane or sevoflurane, but dramatically lower generation of fluoride or other metabolites than any other volatile anaesthetic agent.

6.6 Induction agents

Thiopental has an increased volume of distribution in obese subjects, presumably due to its lipid solubility. Plasma protein binding is largely unchanged. As a consequence of this, although its clearance is the same as in lean individuals, there is a prolonged terminal elimination half-life. A dose for induction of anaesthesia of 7.5 mg per kilogram ideal body weight has been proposed.

Propofol is used both as an induction and as a maintenance agent. It is attractive in the obese population for both purposes. Several studies have suggested that the induction dose of anaesthesia with propofol should be calculated based on ideal body weight. However, the studies on propofol are somewhat conflicting. Some data have suggested that, following a fixed rate infusion of propofol, plasma concentrations are dependent on total body weight. This implies that there is accumulation of propofol in obese subjects. Other studies dispute this, and suggest that propofol target controlled infusion can be based on either total body weight or corrected weight, without modification of the infusion algorithm. The cautious clinical approach would be to use propofol target controlled infusion for anaesthesia only where monitoring of depth of anaesthesia (e.g., bispectral index) is available.

Benzodiazepines are highly lipid soluble, and this is associated with an increased volume of distribution in obese subjects. Both the volume of distribution and elimination half-time of midazolam increase proportionately with total body weight. These findings are consistent with an unchanged clearance in obese subjects. This implies that midazolam should be administered in a greater absolute dose (an uncorrected milligrams per kilogram dose) to achieve the same effect-site concentration as in lean individuals. The increased volume of distribution means that the larger absolute dose results in a prolonged duration of action. It has been suggested that, when midazolam is used as a continuous infusion, this should be tailored to the ideal body weight rather than total body weight.

6.7 Opioid agents

The commonly used opioids in the anaesthetic practice (particularly the fentanyl series) are highly lipophilic. In principle, these drugs have a substantially increased volume of distribution and a prolonged elimination half-life in obese patients. Clinical studies have not always been able to confirm this. Data relating to the pharmacokinetics of fentanyl have failed to detect any clinically relevant difference between obese and non-obese subjects. Alfentanil has been studied both as a bolus drug and as an agent for infusion. Obesity seems to have no effect on alfentanil clearance, but does have an important effect on its volume of distribution and especially on the size of the central compartment. Hence, total body weight is appropriate in dose calculations relating to alfentanil.

There are conflicting results regarding sufentanil: in some studies, it behaves similarly in both obese and non-obese subjects, whereas in others, it exhibits an increased volume of distribution and terminal elimination half-life, correlating with body mass index. On balance, it seems likely that, as body mass index rises, sufentanil shows an increased volume of distribution through both lean and adipose compartments.

Remifentanil, despite theoretical similarities in terms of its high lipid solubility, is infused according to lean body mass. This may be because it is very rapidly metabolised by plasma cholinesterases, and therefore has relatively little opportunity for significant redistribution into secondary and tertiary compartments.

There has been much interest recently in the use of paracetamol (acetaminophen) for perioperative analgesia. This resurgence of interest has been largely prompted by the recent clinical availability of a parenteral preparation of paracetamol. Current data suggest that the volume of distribution is related primarily to the size of the central compartment. There is, however, an increased clearance of paracetamol in obese subjects. In clinical practice, these data mean that a standard dose (either in milligrams per kilogram ideal body weight or an unmodified bolus dose of 1 g) is appropriate to achieving therapeutic plasma concentrations. An increase in the dose may result in toxic concentrations. However, the increased clearance and hence shorter half-life means that more frequent dosing with paracetamol may be appropriate in the obese.

6.8 Neuromuscular blocking drugs

The majority of non-depolarising neuromuscular blocking agents are moderately lipophilic drugs. On this basis, they are generally administered according to a corrected body weight. The value used for calculation of dose is the ideal body weight plus 20% of the excess. However, there is a huge inter-individual variability.

In the case of atracurium, the published data are conflicting. Some studies have suggested that the duration of action is entirely independent of relative compartment size, and that total body weight is appropriate for dose calculations in all cases. Other studies have failed to confirm this. The authors' own clinical experience is that the variability between different individuals is huge, and that it is difficult to make predictions either on the effect of a bolus dose or its duration based purely on body weight. Functional monitoring of neuromuscular blockade using a nerve simulator is mandatory.

There are relatively few data published regarding *cis*-atracurium. The limited data suggest that a dose administered on the basis of total body weight results in a similar onset of action and degree of neuromuscular blockade, but a prolonged duration of action. Similar data have been published for rocuronium. A dose based on total body weight gives rapid intubating conditions, but a prolonged duration of action; a dose based on ideal body weight gives delayed and poorer intubating conditions, but a standard duration of action.

The dose of suxamethonium (and theoretically of mivacurium) should be based on total body weight, as this yields best intubating conditions. The offset of action is a function of cholinesterase activity, which is increased in morbidly obese subjects in-line with the increase in total body weight.

6.9 **Conclusions**

Although there are complex pharmacodynamic and pharmacokinetic considerations, which predict the likely behaviour of drugs in the obese, variability between individuals is so great that these predictions are often of very limited clinical value. Judicious drug administration, together with functional monitoring (BIS score, neuromuscular block monitoring), represents the safest approach. For some drugs, relatively robust data exist. However, the appropriate type of body weight on which to base dosing calculations (total body weight, lean body mass, ideal body weight) depends on the compartmental distribution of the individual drug. In many cases, theoretical behaviour and experimental data are poorly correlated.

Further reading

Bouillon T, Shafer SL (1998). Does size matter? *Anesthesiology* **89**(3): 557–60.

Casati A, Putzu M (2005). Anesthesia in the obese patient: pharmacokinetic considerations. *J Clin Anesth* **17**(2): 134–45.

Eger EI II, Saidman LJ (2005). Illustrations of inhaled anesthetic uptake, including intertissue diffusion to and from fat. *Anesth Analg* **100**(4): 1020–33.

Gepts E (1998). Pharmacokinetic concepts for TCI anaesthesia. *Anaesthesia* **53**(Suppl 1): 4–12.

Chapter 7

Pre-operative assessment and preparation

> **Key points**
> - Few pre-operative assessment guidelines are specific to obesity.
> - The purposes of pre-operative assessment are to improve the quality of care and maximise efficient use of theatre time.
> - Anaesthetists carry an overall responsibility for pre-operative assessment.
> - In preassessment protocols, morbidly obese patients should be allocated to a higher ASA grade than history alone suggests.
> - An anaesthetist experienced in treating morbidly obese patients should be involved in pre-operative assessment.

7.1 Organisational considerations

Numerous documents and guidelines have been produced relating to pre-operative assessment. Very few are specific to obesity, and many fail to mention obesity at all. Therefore, local guidelines and protocols need to be developed and implemented. Ideally, these could be logged on a central database so that different departments and institutions could work from a common core of principles. This would lead to an improvement in the quality of pre-operative assessment of the obese patient, together with uniformity of practice, best use of resource, and rapid implementation of new evidence as it becomes available. Such an approach is likely to improve quality of care and improve safety for this high-risk patient population.

The purpose of pre-operative assessment is not only to improve the quality of care and reduce the risk of anaesthesia and surgery to the patient, but also to maximise efficient use of theatre time, for example, by ensuring that all necessary drugs, equipments, and other resources are available prior to commencement of the procedure.

Pre-operative assessment allows identification of those patients likely to need special perioperative care, or who are likely to require post-operative management in a high dependency or critical care environment. This facilitates planning the clinical service.

Anaesthetists carry an overall responsibility for the pre-operative assessment and preparation of patients whom they anaesthetise. This responsibility is often delegated, for example, to a nurse-led pre-assessment clinic, or to another anaesthetist (not necessarily the doctor who is going to administer anaesthesia to the patient).

When obese patients present for emergency surgery, there is relatively little time for pre-operative preparation. The assessment, in this situation, is clinically based and should take account of the results of basic investigations. These should include full blood count, electrolytes, renal and hepatic function, ECG, and chest X-ray. It is unlikely that further or complex investigations can be obtained in the emergency. Furthermore, the risk attributable to lack of investigations has to be balanced against the risk of delaying surgery.

Key points in the assessment of the obese patient presenting for emergency surgery are similar to those for elective surgery. These relate primarily to the airway, fluid balance, and to the cardiovascular and respiratory systems. It may be necessary to delay surgery to allow appropriate fluid resuscitation and respiratory support, for example, chest physiotherapy, nebulisers, or perioperative continuous positive airway pressure (CPAP). Baseline arterial blood gases should be performed whenever possible. Appropriate staffing, theatre, and perioperative resources must also be made available, despite short notice.

Obese and morbidly obese patients often suffer significant and multiple co-morbidities. These can have a significant impact on the practical conduct of anaesthesia, and may require further investigation or elucidation before a safe and appropriate anaesthetic plan can be developed. Patients presenting for elective surgery should undergo full pre-operative assessment and preparation. Some patients are admitted for elective surgery the day prior to operation, allowing limited time for preassessment. The majority are likely to be admitted on the day of surgery, having previously attended an outpatient pre-assessment clinic. This allows time for pre-operative assessment and planning. Morbidly obese patients should be fully preassessed, even when scheduled for minor procedures.

A visit to an appropriately set up outpatient pre-operative assessment clinic allows time for a proper and full evaluation of the patient's condition and likely perioperative requirements. Further tests and investigations can be organised as necessary. When the results of these are available, the patient can be offered a clear explanation of the proposed plan of treatment. This allows the patient a suitable opportunity to ask questions about his/her anaesthetic. Appropriate use of an outpatient-preassessment facility in this way is valuable to the hospital as well as to the patient, as it allows for planning of appropriate staffing and a balanced case-mix for the operating session. This is economically valuable to the hospital, and can justify the cost of running a pre-operative assessment clinic.

This point is emphasised by the pre-operative assessment guidelines published by the Association of Anaesthetists of Great Britain and Ireland (2001). This guideline sets out good practice for pre-operative assessment, and states that hospitals and anaesthetic departments 'should ensure that the necessary time and resources are directly targeted towards preoperative assessment'. Other countries have similar guidelines. In Belgium, for example, there are 'Safety First Guidelines'.

Algorithms for pre-operative patient assessment are complex. The NICE guidelines for pre-operative assessment provide tables of appropriate investigations according to defining categories. NICE do not include obesity as a defining category in their look-up tables. Rather, the tables are based on the age of the patient and the magnitude of the surgical procedure (classified from one to four in order of increasing severity, with separate additional categories for cardiac and neuro-surgery). Separate tables are produced according to ASA status and the presence of major organ system co-morbidities.

Local protocols for pre-operative assessment and preparation of obese subjects can be based on NICE guidelines provided a convention is adopted which defines the minimum ASA status of obese, morbidly obese, and super obese subjects. Expert opinion polled during development of the NICE guidelines implied that neither obesity nor smoking was relevant independent clinical factors in patients who would otherwise be categorised as ASA 1. This seems a reasonable position in the case of simple obesity, but should not be extended to include morbidly obese and super obese individuals, who, even in the absence of a history of cardiovascular or respiratory co-morbidity, are at increased perioperative risk. For purposes of preassessment protocols, morbidly obese and super obese patients are better classified to a higher ASA grade than a health history alone would suggest.

NICE guidelines also set out a framework for selection and review of appropriate investigations. They define which investigations are most appropriate, and suggest that investigations should not be performed if they are unlikely to be reviewed by a clinician capable of interpreting them appropriately. Likewise, there should be an appropriate evidence base for changing treatment on the basis of the results of an investigation. Where this does not exist, it is not in the patient's interest for the investigation. A recent Italian study showed that the use of a protocol-driven preassessment schema resulted in a dramatic reduction in tests ordered and a 50% cost saving without detriment to quality of care.

By this argument, one of the most commonly 'over performed' investigations is chest radiography. A chest X-ray is unlikely to be helpful in simple obesity, in the absence of other co-morbidities. However, it becomes increasingly useful, whether as a diagnostic tool or as a baseline with which to compare perioperative and post-operative changes, as ASA status, and body mass index rise.

7.2 Special considerations

A number of special considerations apply when assessing the obese patient prior to anaesthesia. These can be considered both in terms of organisational issues around management of the morbidly obese patient, or in terms of an organ system/co-morbidity-based approach to the problems encountered in the perioperative period.

In order to minimise unnecessary or uninformative special investigations, careful attention should be paid to history and examination. An anaesthetist experienced in treating morbidly obese patients should be involved in the pre-operative assessment, as this may help focus special investigations on those areas likely to affect patient management. Special investigations are important not only to detect positive findings, but also to confirm significant negative findings.

7.3 Cardiovascular system

Particular attention should be paid to the cardiovascular system. A history of chest pain or breathlessness is extremely important. Drug history may also be informative. Presence of oedema or crepitations may suggest right or left heart failure, respectively. Many obese and morbidly obese patients suffer moderate or severe hypertension. There is a relatively high prevalence of ischaemic heart disease, and of altered lipid profiles. Simple cardiovascular history may fail to elicit symptoms, as lifestyle changes and inability to exercise may mask ischaemic heart disease. In addition to basic clinical examination, ECG is mandatory. Patients in whom this is suggestive of ischaemia, or who have a history of ischaemic heart disease, may require further specialist investigation. This may mandate a cardiology referral.

Trans-thoracic cardiac echo in the morbidly obese is often uninformative, as adequate views are often impossible to obtain. Transoesophageal echocardiography offers a theoretical solution to this problem, but in practice may be unavailable or unfeasible in the awake subject. Functional tests such as Bruce protocol treadmill testing are equally unlikely to be helpful in many morbidly obese subjects due to their inability to exercise to the ischaemic threshold. Alternative tests of cardiac ischaemic threshold have been suggested. These include dobutamine stress echo and dipyridamole thallium scanning. Radionuclide myocardial perfusion scanning may be useful in some subjects. Generally, anti-hypertensive and anti-heart failure treatments are continued throughout the perioperative period. Caution should be exercised in patients taking anti-platelet drugs. Clopidogrel should usually be discontinued 10 days prior to surgery.

7.4 **Respiratory system**

Features in the history and clinical examination highly predictive of perioperative difficulty include asthma (up to 30% of morbidly obese patients), obstructive sleep apnoea (see Chapter 5), the obesity hypoventilation syndrome, or cor pulmonale. Many morbidly obese people are hypoxic at rest, or suffer awake hypercarbia. These lesions may be suspected clinically, but should be defined by blood gas analysis.

Chest X-ray and simple pulmonary function tests such as vital-lography or spirometry may be unhelpful. An ECG suggestive of right heart failure or cor pulmonale is always highly suspicious. Further investigations are indicated. These should include echocardiography, chest X-ray, arterial blood gases, and sleep studies. If significant pulmonary hypertension is suspected (e.g., significant court pulmonale, right ventricular hypertrophy, or estimated elevated pulmonary artery pressure on echocardiography) formal pulmonary artery pressure studies or cardiac catheterisation may be required. A period of treatment with CPAP may be indicated if severe obstructive sleep apnoea, the obesity hypoventilation syndrome, and cor pulmonale are confirmed.

7.5 **Airway**

Assessment and management of the airway is covered in detail in Chapter 9. History and examination are the most important first steps. Patients who fulfil standard (non-obesity) criteria for airway difficulty or difficult intubation are likely to be extremely problematic. In addition to this, there are a significant number of patients who would not be expected to have a 'difficult airway' by standard criteria. Some prove difficult under anaesthesia owing to fatty infiltration of the pharyngeal wall or altered upper airway compliance. This can lead to airway obstruction during anaesthesia. These problems can persist into the post-operative period. Suggestive features in the history and on examination include obstructive sleep apnoea, hyper-carbia at rest, 'snuffling', adenoidal breathing, or 'snoring' while awake. Special investigations include polysomnography and lateral cephalometry. In extreme cases, the airway may be further imaged by magnetic resonance scanning.

7.6 **Renal**

Many morbidly obese patients suffer renal dysfunction or borderline renal failure. This may not represent a primary feature of obesity, but rather a complication of other co-morbidities. These include hypertension and diabetes. Renal dysfunction may also be seen as a consequence of long-term use of non-steroidal anti-inflammatory drugs.

Worsening of renal function is often seen in the perioperative period, potentially because of the syndrome of inappropriate anti-diuretic hormone secretion (SIADH), together with alterations in organ blood flow and the abdominal compartment syndrome. These changes can be further exacerbated by perioperative hypotension and the use of non-steroidal anti-inflammatory drugs for post-operative analgesia.

Clinical experience has shown that most of the patients at risk are the elderly morbidly obese with diabetes, particularly those with baseline renal impairment or proteinuria. Patients in whom these problems are detected pre-operatively require special care and avoidance of non-steroidal anti-inflammatory drugs in the post-operative period.

7.7 **Gastrointestinal system**

High intra-abdominal pressure (associated with the android fat distribution) may be associated with perioperative abdominal compartment syndrome and an increased risk of oesophageal reflux. Fatty liver, hepatic fibrosis, and cirrhosis may also be seen in this group of patients, but are frequently difficult to detect on the basis of pre-operative history and examination. In some cases, liver function tests or clotting may be disturbed, but these tend to be late changes. Because there is substantial functional reserve, deterioration of liver synthetic function does not manifest in altered blood tests until there is a loss of around 85% of hepatocyte mass.

Symptoms or signs of reflux, asthma, early morning wheeziness, or tight chest all constitute an adequate clinical indication for pre-operative prescription of antacid drugs. H_2 blockers, pro-kinetic drugs, and proton pump inhibitors are all widely used in clinical practice. There is a strong case for using one or more of these classes of drugs routinely in all obese patients presenting for surgery. Patients with a strongly suggestive history should be considered either for a rapid sequence induction of anaesthesia or and awake incubation.

In some cases, a regional anaesthetic technique may be possible and may circumvent these issues.

7.8 Metabolic derangement

The principal metabolic derangements encountered include altered lipid profiles, diabetes (often with insulin resistance), and fatty liver. Many morbidly obese patients suffer hypothyroidism, or are treated with thyroxine for a presumed state of relative hypothyroidism. Consideration needs to be given to therapy of these conditions in the perioperative period. Drugs such as statins and thyroxine should be continued throughout the perioperative period wherever possible, with minimal disruption of the normal dosing regimen.

Oral anti-diabetic drugs should not be given on the day of surgery because of the risk of intra-operative hypoglycaemia. Metformin should be discontinued at least 24 h before surgery, not only because of the risk of perioperative hypoglycaemia, but also because of the increased incidence of lactic acidosis seen in patients taking this drug. In some cases, introduction of an insulin sliding scale regimen may be helpful. Because of insulin resistance seen in many morbidly obese patients, perioperative glucose control may prove problematic.

7.9 Locomotor system

Attention should be given to the musculoskeletal and locomotor systems. Many patients suffer reduced mobility as a consequence of arthritis and other obesity-related co-morbidities. Consequently, they may be taking specific drugs, including non-steroidal anti-inflammatory agents, other analgesics, or anti-arthritic drugs that have the potential to cause drug interactions ought other complications in the perioperative period. Musculoskeletal problems also have direct implications for perioperative patient positioning as well as for post-operative pain relief. These issues should be adequately explored at pre-operative assessment, and any decisions/strategies for perioperative care documented in the anaesthetic plan.

7.10 Psychological preparation

This may be particularly relevant in patients presenting for bariatric surgery. In an Australasian series of patients presenting for bariatric surgery, all assessed by a single psychiatrist, only one serves were completely straightforward: 58% had some identifiable psychiatric morbidity and 9% were excluded from the programme because of doubtful motivation. Morbidly obese patients often suffer a range of co-morbidities, and it is not surprising that some of these are psychiatric. Appropriate assessment, reassurance, and perioperative support should be in place (this includes patient support groups and self-help communities).

7.11 Conclusions

Pre-operative assessment should be performed in all patients. There are few specific algorithms published for pre-operative assessment of the morbidly obese. This patient group stands to derive great benefit from timely pre-operative assessment. Secondary advantages and benefits include improved organisation and efficiency to support the needs of the morbidly obese patient, and of the clinical team, at the time of surgery.

Protocols may need to be constructed locally so that appropriate pre-operative assessment can be effectively and efficiently provided for obese patients. National and international pre-operative assessment guidelines include relatively little guidance specifically tailored to the obese. The preassessment process for the morbidly obese patient should be overseen by an appropriately skilled and experienced anaesthetist. This anaesthetist should be directly involved in delivery of the patient's subsequent anaesthetic.

Further reading

Ferrando A, Ivaldi C, Buttiglieri A, Pagano E, Bonetto C, Arione R, Scaglione L, Gelormino E, Merletti F, Ciccone G (2005). Guidelines for preoperative assessment: impact on clinical practice and costs. *Int J Qual Health Care* **17**(4): 323–9.

Fischer, SP (1996). Development and effectiveness of an anesthesia preoperative evaluation clinic in a teaching hospital. *Anesthesiology* **85**(1): 196–206.

Gertler R, Ramsey-Stewart G (1986). Pre-operative psychiatric assessment of patients presenting for gastric bariatric surgery (surgical control of morbid obesity). *Aust N Z J Surg* **56**(2): 157–61.

National Collaborating Centre for Acute Care. The use of routine preoperative tests for elective surgery. London: National Institute for Health and Clinical Excellence, (2003). http://www.nice.org.uk/guidance/CG3

Preoperative assessment: the role of the anaesthetist. London: Association of Anaesthetists of Great Britain and Ireland, (2001). http://www.aagbi.org/publications/guidelines.htm

Chapter 8

Practical conduct of anaesthesia and the anaesthetic environment

> ### Key points
>
> - Safe practical conduct of anaesthesia for the morbidly obese, whether by a regional or general anaesthetic technique, requires an appropriately equipped operating theatre or other anaesthetic environment.
> - Sufficient staff must be available throughout the anaesthetic period to assist with handling and positioning the patient.
> - A dedicated operating theatre, an equipment checklist, or 'obesity pack' may be extremely helpful in organising the clinical service.
> - Morbidly obese patients experience a high complication rate, so maximum notice is required so that staff of appropriate experience and seniority are in attendance.

Safe provision of anaesthesia and surgery for morbidly obese patients requires an integrated multidisciplinary approach. Appropriate skills and training are needed by all members of the team. Morbidly obese patients may be too large or too heavy for standard equipment to be used. They have a higher prevalence of co-morbidity, and a higher risk of perioperative complications and problems. The 'anaesthetic environment' must therefore be adequately prepared and equipped against all contingencies.

8.1 The anaesthetic environment

The range of special equipment needed is unlikely to be available in every site throughout the hospital where anaesthetics may be given. Organisationally, it is appropriate that an operating theatre is designated for use as the 'morbid obesity' theatre. This means that special equipment can be concentrated at one location. It may not be organisationally feasible for all morbidly obese patients to be treated at this location. For example, there may be occasions when morbidly obese patients require anaesthesia in 'outside areas', including CT scanners, vascular radiology suites, or day case units.

To streamline the process, and to forestall unforeseen problems, it has been recommended that all hospitals have an 'obesity team'. In large hospitals with a bariatric surgery programme, this would be the bariatric theatre team, but could be others who have the experience of managing morbidly obese patients. In smaller hospitals, key individuals should be nominated to take a lead role in training and service provision.

An 'obesity pack' is a useful approach to managing the occasional morbidly obese patient presenting out with the habitual environment and team. This may take the form of a collection of equipment which can be readily moved from site to site, or can be a 'virtual pack', comprising appropriate information and checklists so that theatre staff can ensure that necessary equipment is available at the site where it is required. In many cases, some, but not all, of the existing equipment may be perfectly adequate, and the information in the obesity pack serves to confirm this prior to the patient's arrival. Supplementary equipment can be obtained according to the pack.

Items which may need to be verified prior to treating a morbidly obese patient include theatre trolleys and operating tables. The maximum safe weight rating varies according to the piece of equipment. More modern equipment is generally rated to a higher weight than older equipment. Typical weight ratings for operating tables range from 130 kg upwards. Similar weight ratings apply to hospital beds. Many modern beds have hydraulic mechanisms for positioning patients more conveniently, for example, moving the patient automatically into a semi-sitting position. Similarly, pneumatic mattresses usually have a 'cardiac arrest' facility. When this is deployed, pneumatic support is lost so that pulmonary resuscitation may be more effectively performed. Devices of this nature are relatively easy to overload if the patient is too heavy. As many morbidly obese patients weigh in excess of 200 kg, this presents a genuine practical problem. In the authors' own hospital, there have been incidents where automated equipment of this nature has failed under the weight of super obese patients. This may render care in the perioperative period extremely difficult, and could potentially lead to patient harm.

An important example of this problem relates to radiology suites. The automated tables in many radiology suites are designed for loads only to 130 kg. Although there is some redundancy in most tolerances, X-ray tables may have to slide out to relatively extreme positions. The author has direct experience of a super obese patient undergoing a CT scan where weight-related equipment failure complicated the procedure. The patient became semi-wedged in the scanner ring, and attempts to dislodge him proved difficult as the sliding table, at full extension, was overloaded and its mechanism failed. Fortunately, manual operation was possible.

Because of the risk of problems of this nature, it is important not to exceed specified weight ratings for theatre and radiology department equipment. This may preclude super obese patients from radiological procedures or interventions. There are anecdotal reports of super obese patients being transferred to a veterinary hospital to be scanned through equipment designed for racehorses. Clearly, the increasing prevalence of morbid obesity has important implications for the future design of radiological and operating theatre equipment.

Patient transfer to and from the operating theatre is often best accomplished on the patient's bed, rather than on an operating theatre trolley. Theatre trolleys are often too narrow to accommodate morbidly obese patients either safely or comfortably. Special obesity-rated beds are available. Larger hospitals with a bariatric surgery programme usually own such beds and are familiar with limitations in their use. Other hospitals hire obesity-rated beds on the basis of clinical need. However, these may not be of standard dimensions, and therefore it is important to confirm that they can pass easily through a hospital corridors and doorways. Although in principle hospital access routes are designed according to appropriate specifications, in practice, particularly in older buildings, there may be restricted access.

Beds used to transport patients to and from the operating room need to be equipped with appropriate monitoring, oxygen cylinders, and portable continuous positive airway pressure (CPAP). An equipment rack may need to be fitted to accommodate such devices. On arrival in the operating theatre, the patient is transferred to the operating table and monitoring is instituted. The transfer may be problematic. Some patients can position themselves on the operating table. In other situations, this may not be possible, so sufficient staff and appropriate equipments are needed to move the patient.

A number of devices have been used for this purpose. Simplest is the 'Pat slide' device, a low friction board which can be placed under the patient so that the theatre team can more easily slide the patient from the bed to the operating table. Such devices are not appropriate for patients at the heavier end of the range. For this group, mechanical hoists can be used. A practical and successful alternative is the hover mattress. This is a low friction bag placed under the patient, which is connected to an air pump allowing it to be inflated. It then behaves as the skirts of a Hovercraft, allowing the patient to be moved almost effortlessly between bed and table.

8.2 **Conduct of anaesthesia**

Once positioned on the table, the patient is encouraged to feel for the edges of the table, as operating tables are narrower than the patient's bed. It is important the patient is appropriately centred or positioned for subsequent surgery. If the proposed operation requires the patient in a lateral position, it may be best for the patient to assume this position while awake. Anaesthesia can be induced in the lateral position. If this option is chosen, it is important that the anaesthetist is familiar with managing and intubating a patient on his/her side. In practice, this is relatively straightforward, particularly when the patient is positioned on his left. If the patient is to be positioned on his right, a reverse blade laryngoscope is required. Oxygenation is likely to be better with the patient in a lateral position because of the reduced effects of abdominal compression on functional residual capacity.

For patients who are placed in the supine position, it is generally appropriate for the operating table to be positioned with a head up tilt between 15° and 25°. At this stage, relevant monitoring equipments can be connected. At a minimum, this includes pulse oximetry, ECG, and blood pressure monitoring. If this is to be done by cuff manometer, a large cuff is needed. A ratio between arm circumference and cuff breadth of 1:3 has been suggested. In many heavier patients, non-invasive blood pressure measurement is misleading or inaccurate. Consideration should be given to direct arterial pressure monitoring. A radial artery cannula can be sited before induction of anaesthesia. Even in the largest patients, this is usually relatively straightforward as the artery is readily palpable. In some cases, ultrasound guided radial artery puncture represents a fallback option. Occasionally, it may be necessary to cannulate a brachial artery. Femoral artery puncture is generally undesirable because of hygiene issues.

Thromboprophylaxis is a key issue in the perioperative management of the morbidly obese. In addition to low molecular weight heparin administered pre-operatively, intra-operative and post-operative measures include the use of support stockings or of active calf compression. This option is appropriate in all but most of the minor cases. Calf compression devices, for example, 'Flowtron boots' of a size appropriate to the patient should be fitted and switched on prior to induction of anaesthesia. There are occasions when the compression boots are not large enough to fit around the patient's calves. A pragmatic solution is to use two boots around each calf, joined by Velcro to increase the maximum girth accommodated.

8.3 Vascular access

Gaining appropriate vascular access may prove difficult. A large bore peripheral venous cannula should be inserted where possible. The dorsum of the hand and flexor aspect of the forearm represent the easiest sites for cannulation. Ultrasound has been described as a useful technique for gaining peripheral vascular access in morbidly obese patients. Where large bore peripheral access is not possible, central venous access via the internal jugular route, under ultrasound guidance, represents a feasible alternative.

If central venous access cannulation is to be attempted, the patient should be positioned supine with the head turned to the contralateral side. Supplementary oxygen should be administered at this stage. After an explanation of the procedure, an assistant retracts the soft tissues of the chest away from the patient's neck using the flat of the hand. This allows adequate access for the ultrasound probe, and for cannulation of the internal jugular vein.

When ultrasound is not available, or in emergency, a blind approach may be attempted. A useful technique for this is the 'very high' approach. In this approach, the operator's fingertips are used to identify the groove between the mandible and the sternomastoid muscle just below the earlobe. The cannulating needle is introduced at a steep angle in this groove, and directed downwards and slightly towards the midline. The internal jugular vein should be encountered before the vertebra is met, and a guide wire passed. The commonest reason for difficulty is excessively lateral puncture.

8.4 Induction of anaesthesia

It is only safe to proceed to induction of anaesthesia when sufficient staff are present to help move or turn the patient in the event of difficulty. Everyone is given clear instructions relating to their role and the importance of remaining in theatre until released. A range of equipments for potential airway problems must be available. The choice between awake or asleep intubation depends on airway, respiratory, and cardiovascular factors, as well as the skills and experience of the anaesthetic team. These issues are discussed more elaborately in Chapter 9.

The risk of reflux and aspiration of gastric contents is theoretically quite high in morbidly obese patients undergoing general anaesthesia. In practice, these risks can be minimised by the use of appropriate pre-medication. Histamine 2 antagonist drugs, proton pump inhibitors, and agents to promote gastric emptying such as metoclopramide all have a role. Benzodiazepine and mild sedative drugs may also be helpful; however, opiate pre-medication should be avoided, both because of the risk of respiratory depression in the perioperative period, and because of reduced gastric emptying which theoretically increases the chances of reflux and aspiration. An individual clinical decision whether modification of the anaesthetic induction technique is warranted has to be made on the balance of risks.

Specific drugs and induction techniques are determined by patient physiology and co-morbidity. Appropriate choices of agents and drug doses have been discussed in Chapter 6. Because of the risk of haemodynamic decompensation, it is appropriate to induce anaesthesia in a cautious and gentle fashion, generally with a fast running intravenous infusion in progress. Although seldom used, a selection of cardiovascular support drugs, including a vasopressor and a beta-blocker, should be available and drawn up in anticipation.

Following induction of anaesthesia, further appropriate monitoring may be instituted. This should include measurement of temperature as well as neuromuscular function. Continuous monitoring of respiratory mechanics and depth of consciousness is desirable. Techniques such as bispectral index monitoring (BIS) are valuable at this stage, because of the variability of effect-site concentration of drugs in obesity.

Logically, the use of short-acting drugs seems attractive, as these are less likely to result in accumulation. Agents such as propofol, desflurane, and sevoflurane have all been advocated for use in the morbidly obese patient. There is a body of evidence to support their use. Combined with shorter acting opioids and neuromuscular blocking agents, a favourable recovery profile is more likely.

Final patient positioning should take account of protection of the skin and pressure points. This can be difficult, particularly where arm boards, retractors, and splints are fitted to table side rails. The dimensions may be narrower than those of the patient.

During the course of surgery, it is important to keep the patient as warm as possible. This reduces post-operative shivering, a cause of hypoxia, neurohumoral stress response, and myocardial ischaemia. Patients can be kept warm intra-operatively by a number of strategies. These include forced warm air over blankets, an isothermic theatre environment, and fluid warmers. In addition to the prevention of post-operative shivering, active patient warming reduces the incidence of post-operative wound infection.

Intra-operative fluids should be carefully titrated to the patient's needs. Fluid should be given to replace blood loss together with a sufficient volume to replace insensible losses and satisfy baseline requirements. Insensible losses are proportional to body surface area. As this value is substantially increased in the obese patient population, absolute volumes of fluid may seem high, even in those patients who are subject to relative fluid restriction.

Excessive fluid loading should be avoided in patients with peripheral oedema, right heart failure, cor pulmonale, or pulmonary hypertension. Equally, those with significant ischaemic heart disease or left ventricular failure are at high risk. Functional fluid responsiveness represents an attractive approach to managing fluid balance (optimisation of stroke volume or fluid titration according to pulse pressure variation). Such techniques guide fluid management more appropriately than simple estimation of central venous pressure.

8.5 Recovery from general anaesthesia

Emergence from general anaesthesia should be carefully managed. It is important to maintain oxygenation and minimise cardiovascular stress at this stage. The risk of hypoxia and aspiration of gastric contents is as high during extubation as it is at induction of anaesthesia. Whenever possible, the patient should be extubated awake in a controlled fashion. After major surgery, this is likely to be in the intensive care unit after a period of elective post-operative ventilation. After lesser procedures, the patient may be extubated in the operating theatre, with enough members of staff present to deal with potential problems, including re-intubation should this be required. The trachea should not be extubated until the patient is fully awake and in control of the airway, and has re-established protective reflexes. The patient should be appropriately positioned for extubation, either in the lateral position or in the fall sitting position where this is possible. He should be able to generate adequate tidal volumes and demonstrate a clinically satisfactory respiratory pattern prior to removal of the endotracheal tube.

A recruitment manoeuvre performed at the time of extubation may help reduce post-operative atelectasis and improve subsequent respiratory function. The use of respiratory stimulant drugs such as doxapram, in judicious doses, has a rationale, as it has been shown to reduce post-operative atelectasis. Successful re-establishment of tidal breathing occurs once the depressant effects of anaesthetic and analgesic drugs have tailed off. A sufficiently high arterial/brain partial pressure of carbon dioxide is required. There is a risk of hypoventilation and atelectasis development while the carbon dioxide tension is rising to this critical value. Following extubation, it may be necessary to apply the facial CPAP immediately, to employ a nasopharyngeal airway, or both. The patient should then be transferred to a suitable environment for observation during the recovery period.

8.6 **Regional anaesthesia**

Regional anaesthetic techniques seem particularly attractive in the morbidly obese patient. When these are performed, they can avoid many of the risks of general anaesthesia. In particular, the patient is able to maintain his own airway, and is not subject to many of the disorders of respiratory control associated with general anaesthesia. However, these 'advantages' are lost, and greater disadvantages may accrue if it becomes necessary to convert to a general anaesthetic (failed block, inadequate duration, patient positioning, or discomfort). Similarly, advantages may be limited in the case of neuraxial blockade, which causes sympathetic nervous system and respiratory muscle involvement. This can result in perioperative atelectasis, shunt, and hypoxia, even in the fully awake patient.

A number of problems attend regional anaesthesia in morbidly obese subjects. It may be technically more difficult to perform the block in this patient group. Especially long needles may be required, particularly for sub-arachnoid and epidural anaesthesia. Successful central block has been described using a 120 mm needle in the super obese obstetric population.

Blocks should only be performed by those proficient in them and who perform them regularly. Difficulty palpating landmarks and defining surface anatomy for performance of regional blocks may present a major challenge. The availability of good-quality ultrasound equipment can to some extent help overcome this problem. Indeed, ultrasound guided regional anaesthesia has recently been hailed as the gold standard.

8.7 **Emergency surgery**

Patients presenting for emergency procedures should be assessed and considered in much the same way as those presenting for elective surgery. There is a shorter time available for pre-operative preparation. Such patients may suffer fluid and electrolyte disturbances, and potentially have a full stomach. These factors should be taken into account when planning the anaesthetic. The operating theatre team should be given as much warning as possible of the morbidly obese emergency patient, so that appropriate equipments and staffing can be put in place. Consideration needs to be given to the choice of location and monitoring in the post-operative period. Even after minor surgery, the combination of a morbidly obese patient, emergency surgery, and the short time available for preparation and optimisation make post-operative high dependency care desirable.

8.8 **Obstetric anaesthesia**

There is an increasing prevalence of obesity in pregnant women. Figures from the United States in the past 10 years have placed this between 18.5 and 38.3%. European data suggest that, for women in the reproductive age group, the prevalence reached 18.3% in 2002. Because obesity results in an increased perinatal risk, obese parturient women should have an anaesthetic assessment during their pregnancy.

Physiological changes in pregnancy interact with the physiological changes of obesity to enhance risk. The cardiovascular changes of pregnancy (associated with an increased oxygen demand) combine with those of obesity to produce increased cardiovascular stress. This is to some extent offset by pregnancy-induced changes in the respiratory system, which counteract those of obesity. Although both pregnancy and obesity result in reduced functional residual capacity, there are improvements in carbon dioxide sensitivity and respiratory control from early pregnancy onwards, which protect against sleep apnoea and the obesity hypoventilation syndrome.

The combined effects of obesity and pregnancy on maternal physiology can be very detrimental. There are reported cases of sudden cardiovascular death when obese pregnant women adopt the supine position. Furthermore, the combined effects of endothelial dysfunction seen in both pregnancy and obesity result in an increased prevalence of pregnancy-related hypertension and pre-eclampsia. The incidence of other complications is also greater in pregnant women who are obese; these include diabetes, asthma, and thromboembolic disease. Not surprisingly, there is not only increased maternal morbidity and mortality in pregnancy, but also increased foetal morbidity. Both foetal death and birth defects are more common in maternal obesity.

A regional anaesthetic is therefore even more desirable in the obese parturient than in others. Single-shot sub-arachnoid block has been quoted as the most popular technique. However, using a narrow gauge spinal needle to identify the sub-arachnoid space presents considerable technical challenges in the obese. Placing an epidural catheter may be technically easier. Some authorities have advocated routine prophylactic siting of an epidural catheter in all labouring obese mothers so that subsequent analgesia or conversion to caesarean section can be performed more easily and safely.

Obese mothers have a higher rate of operative delivery and of caesarean section than non-obese individuals. The perioperative complication rate is also higher, with infection and thromboembolic phenomena high up on the list.

8.9 **Laparoscopic surgery**

Laparoscopic surgery stresses the respiratory and cardiovascular systems. Most bariatric surgery is performed laparoscopically. Hence, the challenges of the reverse Trendelenberg position are combined with those of pneumoperitoneum and those of upper abdominal surgery. Gynaecological surgery is also frequently performed laparoscopically, but in the steep head down position. In this situation, cardiovascular embarrassment is traded for worse respiratory compromise.

Instillation of carbon dioxide into the peritoneum has clinical and physiological consequences. First, the patient is unlikely to be supine. If the head up position is adopted, then there is reduced venous return and reduced cardiac output as a consequence of venous pooling in the lower limbs. This is further exacerbated by the effects of raised intra-abdominal pressure. This gives rise to a further reduction in venous return, together with splanchnic ischaemia. Depending on the inflation pressure used and the duration of surgery, there may also be passage of gas into the tissues, with development of surgical emphysema. There is progressive elevation of arterial carbon dioxide tension. This results in a respiratory acidosis and activation of the sympathetic nervous system. Tachydysrhythmias may result. There is increased systemic vascular resistance, and arterial pressure is maintained at the expense of cardiac output. These changes also potentially result in increased pulmonary artery pressure, increased intracranial pressure (ICP), and reduced cerebral perfusion. As morbidly obese patients occasionally suffer obesity-related intracranial hypertension, in some cases severe enough to warrant surgical shunting – any procedure likely to elevate ICP further may be deleterious (Table 8.1).

These factors all make invasive monitoring of arterial pressure and good vascular access more important. Ventilation using high inspiratory pressures and positive end expiratory pressure (PEEP) may be necessary to maintain adequate oxygenation. This risks compromising cardiovascular function even further.

8.10 **Day case surgery**

Many obese patients may be suitable for day case anaesthesia, particularly where this is for minor or body surface surgery. Although there is an increased risk of perioperative morbidity which rises in line with body mass index, the patient should not be excluded from day case surgery solely on the basis of body mass index. This is because the increased risk is likely to be small in the case of minor surgery, particularly in those patients who suffer no co-morbidity or only minimal co-morbidity. In many countries, day case surgery is

Table 8.1 Effects of pneumoperitoneum relevant to the morbidly obese patient
Reduced venous return
Reduced cardiac output
Raised intra-abdominal pressure   Splanchnic ischaemia
Migration of gas into the tissues   Development of surgical emphysema
Progressive elevation of arterial carbon dioxide tension   Respiratory acidosis

Activation of sympathetic nervous system
   Tachydysrhythmias
   Increased systemic vascular resistance
   Arterial pressure maintained at the expense of cardiac output

Increased pulmonary artery pressure
Increased intracranial pressure
High inspiratory pressures and PEEP   Further reduction in cardiac output

standard practice even in morbidly obese patients. In the United Kingdom, Department of Health guidelines suggest that it should be the norm in patients up to a body mass index of 40 kgm^{-2}.

When the body mass index exceeds this, the patient should be reviewed in a preassessment clinic by a suitably experienced anaesthetist. In the absence of serious co-morbidity, there is relatively no little good evidence to exclude the patient from the day case programme purely on the basis of body mass index. Indeed, a large clinical series has suggested that otherwise fit patients do not have a clinically higher risk of prolonged hospital stay all major morbidity when treated as day cases as compared to non-obese individuals. It is now common practice to accept all patients for day surgery whose management would be the same whether conducted as an inpatient or as a day case.

Patients may be accepted for day case surgery in the presence of co-morbidity, provided this is stable and is unlikely either to deteriorate as a result of surgery, or to prolong hospital admission. Anaesthetic management of morbidly obese patients may differ from that of lean individuals. For example, morbidly obese patients undergoing day case surgery may require intubation and ventilation to protect the airway and to facilitate adequate gas exchange. In this respect, they may differ from non-obese individuals. This should not, however, preclude day care.

8.11 **Conclusions**

In the majority of studies, morbidly obese patients have consistently demonstrated increased perioperative morbidity and mortality. A major cultural change in our approach to this patient group is required if risk is to be minimised. Safe anaesthesia for the obese patient requires a package of measures, encompassing environment, equipment, expertise, and training not normally available in all anaesthetic situations. Locally developed guidelines can assist in this.

Further reading

Blackshaw R, Peat W, Youngs P (2006). Use of ultrasound to obtain peripheral venous access. *Int J Obstet Anesth* **15**(2): 174–5.

Cevik B, Ilham C, Orskiran A, Colakoglu S (2006). Morbid obesity: a risk factor for maternal mortality. *Int J Obstet Anesth* **15**(3): 263.

Davies KE, Houghton K, Montgomery JE (2001). Obesity and day-case surgery. *Anaesthesia* **56**(11): 1112–5.

Hopkins PM (2007). Ultrasound guidance as a gold standard in regional anaesthesia. *Br J Anaesth* **98**: 299–301.

Nitta R, Yabe M, Sato M, Kimura T, Nishikawa T (2006). Successful epidural anesthesia using 120 mm epidural needle for caesarean section in a morbidly obese parturient with body mass index 50.2 kgm^{-2}. *Masui* **55**(11): 1409–11.

Obesity guideline. London: Association of Anaesthetists of Great Britain and Ireland, (2007). http://www.aagbi.org/publications/guidelines.htm.

Saravanakumar K, Rao SG, Cooper GM (2006). Obesity and obstetric anaesthesia. *Anaesthesia* **61**(1): 36–48.

Chapter 9

Obesity and the airway

Key points

- Airway management in the obese patient is challenging.
- The presence of obstructive sleep apnoea and other obstructive symptoms is highly suggestive of airway difficulty.
- Standard history and examination may fail to predict airway difficulty in the obese.
- Airway obstruction during spontaneous breathing may result from fatty infiltration of the wall of the pharynx, with increased pharyngeal wall compliance.
- Asleep intubation should only be attempted by an experienced anaesthetist with adequate assistance. It is desirable for two anaesthetists to be present.
- Awake intubation may provide a safer alternative to intubation under general anaesthesia.
- Similar considerations and care apply to extubation as to intubation.
- Airway problems continue into the post-operative period.

The anaesthetist faced with a morbidly obese patient may find the airway challenging. A number of features contributed to this challenge. These include both anatomical and pathophysiological disturbances. Anatomically, the patient may be both difficult to ventilate by a face mask and difficult to intubate. Because of body habitus and fat disposition, spontaneous ventilation is seldom an option. It is further limited by the combined risks of hypoventilation, regurgitation and aspiration of gastric contents, and airway obstruction.

Physiologically, the patient is likely to have an increased intra-pulmonary shunt and a reduced functional residual capacity. This means that apnoea results in much more rapid arterial desaturation and onset of profound hypoxaemia then would be the case in a non-obese individual. Computer modelling suggests that, even after highly effective preoxygenation for 5 min, arterial desaturation to critical levels (60% or less) would occur in around 4 min in an obese (120 kg) individual. This is more rapid than the arterial desaturation to be expected in a 10 kg child. Desaturation to critical values is predicted to take around 10 min in a fit 70 kg adult.

These times represent the theoretical times to desaturation, in an ideal situation where preoxygenation has been 'perfect'. Consequently, they somewhat overestimate the margin of safety. In clinical practice, desaturation to critical levels occurs rather more rapidly. If preoxygenation does not proceed for a complete 5 min then desaturation is significantly quicker. Moreover, if there is any leak between the face mask and the patient's face during the period of preoxygenation, then the effective alveolar oxygen tension achieved is substantially less than 1.0. When the alveolar oxygen concentration achieved is only 0.6, the time to critical desaturation is around 2–3 min. This situation can be further exacerbated by the presence of obesity-related co-morbidity or pulmonary pathology.

The implication is that the majority of morbidly obese patients presenting even for relatively minor surgery are likely to require intubation, while at the same time presenting considerable challenges to the anaesthetist who wishes to accomplish this.

Several studies suggest that intubation becomes progressively more difficult with increasing body mass index. In an early series, the incidence of difficult incubation under general anaesthesia was 13%. A more recent series suggests that this figure may be as high as 24%, with up to 8% of patients requiring awake intubation. American data have also confirmed that a short thick neck is predictive of difficult intubation. Both obesity and neck circumference are risk factors for obstructive sleep apnoea; obstructive sleep apnoea is a further predictor of difficult intubation. This may be because of internal narrowing of the airway.

Obstructive sleep apnoea is also associated with airway collapse during spontaneous ventilation, with obstruction both of the posterior naso-pharynx and of the oro-pharynx. This makes face mask ventilation difficult. The combination of these factors should lead to a high index of suspicion and caution when the anaesthetist is faced with a morbidly obese patient.

In the authors own institution, the bariatric surgery programme accepts patients with a body mass index of 40 kgm^{-2} and above. The majority of patients have had a body mass index far exceeding this; nevertheless, in a series of over 1500 cases anaesthetised predominantly by two senior anaesthetists, there has been only one failed intubation (with a safe outcome) and an unexpected difficult intubation rate of below 3%. Nevertheless, around 10% of patients were identified as potential difficulty intubations pre-operatively. This experience may reflect differences between American and European practice. Although there are differences in the absolute numbers of patients with a 'difficult airway', the principles are the same.

9.1 Pre-operative assessment

Pre-operative assessment of the airway includes history, physical examination, and in some cases special investigations such as lateral cephalometry and sleep studies. Standard predictors of difficult intubation such as Mallampati score, thyro-mental, and thyro-hyoid distances frequently fail to predict airway and intubation difficulties associated with obesity. Obesity-related problems may become apparent only at the time of airway manipulation, as they may result from narrowing of the airway due to pharyngeal wall fat deposition, increased compliance of the pharyngeal wall, and a large tongue, which, coupled with reduced airway muscle tone, partially obscures the larynx at intubation. This gives the appearances of a relatively anterior laryngeal position.

Patients who give a history of obstructive sleep apnoea are more likely to present airway problems at the time of anaesthesia. Likewise, those in whom this has been confirmed by polysomnography are at particularly increased risk. Clinically, patients who have a large neck circumference or are coarse in the jowl should raise suspicion. Some very high-risk individuals have a severely compromised airway even when fully awake. During normal speech, they are dyspnoeic and frequently pause to draw breath. They may appear to obstruct their airway or to be snoring while awake. They almost invariably offer a history of severe sleep apnoea. Arterial blood gases, where available, show a significantly elevated partial pressure of carbon dioxide. Where no arterial blood gases are available, it is important to establish an approximate value for the end-tidal carbon dioxide concentration with the patient fully awake. This can be done using a tight fitting face mask and capnography.

Severely afflicted individuals may benefit from further anatomical assessment. This includes lateral cephalometry, which can help define the extent to which soft tissue collapse obstructs the upper airway. In some cases, further airway imaging, such as magnetic resonance scanning, can give a clue to potential intubation problems. Magnetic resonance scanning of the airway is a research tool which is seldom used in clinical practice.

When a patient has been identified as being at high risk of airway problems, it is good practice to explain the risks, and the issues surrounding awake intubation. Early discussion with the patient may help to allay their anxiety, and facilitate the subsequent procedure.

9.2 **Practical considerations**

By the time the patient arrives in the operating theatre, a provisional decision should already have been made regarding optimal intubation technique. In the majority of cases, this will be a 'routine' asleep intubation. This for a number of reasons should be performed in the operating theatre, not in an anaesthetic room or other annexe. First, it is important for the patient to be on a suitable operating table which can be tilted both head up and head down; many theatre trolleys are inappropriate to the weight range encountered in the obese. Second, it is important that intubation is performed in an appropriate environment where there is sufficient room for all necessary staff and helpers to move around freely, should manoeuvres such as turning the patient on their side become necessary. Third, there is no place for the practice of anaesthetising a morbidly obese patient in an anaesthetic room, and then disconnecting them from monitoring and respiratory support to move them to an alternative environment. Delays may be encountered owing to the patient's size, and where desaturation and airway collapse consequent on disconnection from the breathing system are obligate consequences.

When the patient arrives in the operating theatre, it is important that positioning on the operating table is suitable for patient comfort, represents a good position for breathing and oxygenation, and an optimal position for intubation. The traditional supine position is inconvenient and inappropriate in most of these respects. First, supine positioning results in the basal collapse and may result not only in symptoms of breathlessness but also in very significant arterial desaturation. The consequent reduction in functional residual capacity reduces the duration of the safe apnoeic interval. In some cases, there may also be cardiovascular compromise due to aorto-caval compression. The supine position presents practical problems for intubation: the more severely obese the subject, the more likely they are to suffer upward displacement of fat from the shoulders and breast tissue, which forces airway closure and can come to lie around the head and neck (Figure 9.1). The traditional 'sniffing the morning air' position may also be very difficult to achieve. A buffalo hump of fat over the shoulders and neck effectively prevents this.

These problems can in part be overcome by tilting the operating table into a reverse Trendelenberg (head-up) tilt prior to induction of anaesthesia. An angle of 25° is quoted in the literature, although this is a fairly steep tilt which many patients find uncomfortable. In practical terms, a tilt of around 15° is a feasible alternative. This has several beneficial effects. First, several studies have shown that the reverse Trendelenberg tilt is associated with improved oxygenation

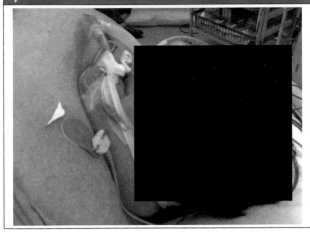

Figure 9.1 Supine position demonstrating airway compromise by torso soft tissues

at the time of induction of anaesthesia, and better preserves functional residual capacity. A secondary advantage is the downward displacement of fatty tissues of the shoulders and upper torso away from the airway. An assistant gently retracting these tissues using the flat of the hand can further aid this.

Instead of pillows or head rings to produce a 'sniffing the morning air' position, a ramp is built using a thin pillow and graduated layers of blankets. The ramp starts at the mid inter-scapular position and increases in depth until the occiput. The ramped head and neck position has been shown to produce substantially better intubating conditions in obese subjects than the traditional intubating position.

If the carbon dioxide partial pressure is not known, it is reasonable to site and arterial line at this stage, and to take a sample for blood gas analysis prior to induction of anaesthesia. Alternatively, a rough estimate can be made based on the end-tidal carbon dioxide measured during preoxygenation. Preoxygenation should be performed with a tight-fitting facemask and a high oxygen fresh gas flow to minimise the risk of entrainment of air between the mask and the face. Many patients prefer to hold the mask themselves. With explanation and a little encouragement, a tight seal can be obtained this way. The application of continuous positive airway pressure (CPAP) (6 cm H_2O) for 5 min in conscious patients has been reported to prevent atelectasis formation during induction of anaesthesia. Furthermore, it improves oxygenation and probably increases the margin of safety before intubation.

Prior to induction of anaesthesia, the final 'pre-flight check' should include a count to ensure that sufficient staff are present to move or turn the patient in the event of difficulty, and that all necessary airway equipment is available to deal with a difficult intubation or a 'can't intubate, can't ventilate' scenario. This should include a full range of laryngoscopes, bougies, and airways, including a range of laryngeal mask airways. Equipment should be available for fibre-optic intubation or emergency crico-thyroidotomy should this be necessary.

In some patients, a history suggestive of reflux makes rapid sequence induction of anaesthesia the technique of choice. In those without a suggestive history, routine induction of anaesthesia followed by facemask ventilation gives stability and controlled intubating conditions. It is desirable to verify that mask ventilation is possible prior to administration of a muscle relaxant.

Ventilation of a morbidly obese patient using a face mask can be technically challenging. In the author's own practice, there are two approaches to this. The first technique involves two anaesthetists to hold the mask, provide forward lift of the jaw, and to ventilate the patient. The second, slightly less cumbersome, technique involves a single anaesthetist holding the face mask in position and displacing the patient's jaw anteriorly using both hands, while ventilation is delivered by a mechanical ventilator. This technique has the advantage that the anaesthetic assistant is free to hand equipment to the anaesthetist, while a second assistant can provide manual retraction of upper torso tissues.

The choice of laryngoscope depends on the experience and preferences of the anaesthetist. A standard blade and handle may be appropriate in some of patients. In most morbidly obese patients, however, the head and neck and chest geometry precludes this. Alternatives include such devices as the polio blade (where the angle between the laryngoscope scope blade and handle is very wide) or the Yentis scope. A number of other innovative solutions have become available in the recent years.

Laryngoscopy may be uncomplicated. In some patients, there is a very narrow field of view owing to fatty infiltration and encroachment of the lateral walls of the airway towards the mid-line. The larynx may appear relatively small and partly obscured by the base of the tongue. An introducer or gum elastic bougie may be necessary at this stage. Confirmation of correct positioning of the endo-tracheal tube by capnography is mandatory.

Following intubation and induction of anaesthesia, ventilation is best continued with addition of positive end expiratory pressure (PEEP). A recent study in patients undergoing bariatric surgery has shown that a recruitment manoeuvre, performed shortly after induction of anaesthesia, has beneficial effects on oxygenation throughout the duration of the case.

9.3 Awake intubation

Awake fibre-optic intubation is the technique of choice when there is any doubt or concern regarding the ease or feasibility of intubation under general anaesthesia. Awake fibre-optic intubation is relatively straightforward in morbidly obese subjects, many of whom have relatively attenuated upper airway reflexes. Most patients tolerate this well, and do not seem to suffer undue stress from the procedure provided suitable explanations and reassurance have been given.

A number of techniques for awake fibre-optic intubation have been described, and there is a wide variety of practice. The most appropriate technique to use is the one with which the anaesthetist is most familiar. A very simple and practical technique involves infusion of low dose remifentanil prior to topical anaesthesia of the airway. The dose chosen will depend on the individual patient, but typically is up to 0.1 µg per kilogram per minute. Once this infusion is established, airway reflexes are further obtunded. Oxygenation should be supported during opioid infusion and attempts at awake intubation. Providing oxygen through a nasal cannula if the oral route is chosen for intubation can do this. Topical anaesthesia of the oropharynx is achieved by judicious spraying with 10% lidocaine topical spray. Anaesthesia of the trachea below the vocal cords can be provided either by using a 'spray as you go' technique or by performing at a trans-cricoid puncture with 3 mL of 2% lidocaine, performed in maximal expiration.

Once adequate topical anaesthesia has been achieved, a 7 mm flexo-metallic tube can easily be railroaded over a fibre-optic intubating scope. Although it is relatively straightforward to do this without any additional equipment, some anaesthetists prefer to use a modified oral airway to stabilise the scope during this manoeuvre. The final position of the tip of the endotracheal tube is confirmed by endoscopy as being in the mid-trachea, well above the carina, and below the vocal cords. The tube is fixed and correct positioning reconfirmed by capnography prior to the induction of anaesthesia.

A number of other techniques are also possible, depending on the skill and experience of the operator.

9.4 Extubation

A number of reports in the literature detail episodes of hypoxia and loss of airway control in the period immediately following extubation. There is no place for extubation of the somnolent or partially awake patient. The choices are between extubation when fully awake and post-operative ventilation.

When awake extubation is chosen, it is important that the patient has an adequate respiratory drive and minute volume prior to extubation. To achieve this, short acting anaesthetic drugs are generally used. It may still be necessary to delay extubation for a considerable time to achieve the necessary preconditions. Ideally, the patient is extubated fully awake and in the sitting position, following a recruitment manoeuvre to limit post-operative atelectasis. An air–oxygen mixture is administered prior to extubation, as either pure oxygen or oxygen with nitrous oxide can result in increased atelectasis, and have the potential to affect post-operative respiratory function adversely. The risk of respiratory depression and airway obstruction continues well into the post-operative period, and is often quoted as persisting up to 7 days.

Patients who are CPAP-dependent at home should bring their machine to hospital with them, as continued use of CPAP throughout the peri-operative period is mandatory. Potentially disastrous deterioration in respiratory function can follow the acute withdrawal of CPAP therapy in the peri-operative period.

9.5 **Conclusions**

Managing the airway in morbidly obese subjects is highly challenging. It requires careful assessment in the pre-operative period, but despite this, unexpected problems can still arise. A full range of difficult airway equipment should always be on hand, as should skilled assistance in the sufficient numbers. In cases of doubt, awake fibreoptic intubation is often the safest option. Difficult airway problems can, and do, continue well into the post-operative period.

Further reading

Benumof JL (2001). Obstructive sleep apnea in the adult obese patient: implications for airway management. *J Clin Anesth* **13**(2): 144–56.

Collins JS, Lemmens HJ, Brodsky JB, Brock-Utne JG, Levitan RM (2004). Laryngoscopy and morbid obesity: a comparison of the 'sniff' and 'ramped' positions. *Obes Surg* **14**(9): 1171–5.

Perilli V, Sollazzi L, Bozza P, Modesti C, Chierichini A, Tacchino RM, Ranieri R (2000). The effects of the reverse trendelenburg position on respiratory mechanics and blood gases in morbidly obese patients during bariatric surgery. *Anesth Analg* **91**(6): 1520–5.

Rusca M, Proietti S, Schnyder P, Frascarolo P, Hedenstierna G, Spahn DR, Magnusson L (2003). Prevention of atelectasis formation during induction of general anesthesia. *Anesth Analg* **97**: 1835–9.

Chapter 10

Recovery and post-operative care

Key points

- Emergence from anaesthesia carries significant risks for the morbidly obese.
- There is a significant risk of hypoxia and loss of control of the airway during the transition from stable anaesthesia to the awake state.
- The anaesthetic technique deployed should be consistent with rapid emergence from anaesthesia and good early airway control.
- Measures of early recovery suggest more rapid emergence from anaesthesia in desflurane-treated patients, but differences have largely disappeared by the time the patient leaves the recovery room.
- A multimodality approach to post-operative analgesia affords good pain relief with least risk of drug side-effects.
- Post-operative intravenous opioids can result in poor post-operative respiratory function.
- Regional anaesthetic techniques can be used for post-operative pain – success can be improved by the use of ultrasound.
- Thoracic epidural anaesthesia is associated with better preservation of respiratory function in the obese as compared with post-operative opiate analgesia.
- Post-operatively, morbidly obese patients should be nursed an appropriate environment.
- If no appropriate post-operative care facility is available, elective surgery should not proceed.

One of the greatest concerns facing the anaesthetist when treating the morbidly obese is the hazard of the recovery phase and immediate post-operative period. Emergence from anaesthesia carries significant risks for the morbidly obese. These relate in particular to airway control, adequacy of respiration (and therefore hypoxia), and post-operative chest complications. In addition to this, there are problems associated with cardiovascular stress and instability.

Post-operative analgesia poses significant challenges in the obese. Many standard techniques are applicable to this patient group, although with special considerations. For example, the obese may be at increased risk of renal dysfunction when treated with non-steroidal anti-inflammatory drugs. There is an increased danger of airway obstruction and respiratory depression associated with opioid agents. Regional blocks may be technically difficult to perform and therefore have an increased failure rate.

A high incidence of post-operative complications, combined with potential difficulties in managing post-operative pain, mean that a simple ward environment may not be appropriate. Many morbidly obese patients undergoing intermediate or major surgery therefore require post-operative admission to a overnight post anaesthetic care unit or high dependency unit.

10.1 **Emergence from anaesthesia**

There is a significant risk of hypoxia and loss of control of the airway during the transition from stable anaesthesia to the awake state. The transition between these two states can be clinically very smooth when the anaesthetic technique has not involved instrumentation of the airway, or when this instrumentation has not been excessively stimulating to the patient. Examples of this included recovery from anaesthesia when a laryngeal mask airway has been used. Low pressure continuous positive airway pressure (CPAP) can be applied to the laryngeal mask airway in the recovery room, and the patient nursed in a semi-recumbent position to maintain oxygenation and maintenance of functional residual capacity. On awakening, the patient removes his own airway. However, laryngeal mask airway anaesthesia in the morbidly obese is limited to a relatively small number of short body surface procedures. Even when it is used in this setting, there is a substantial conversion rate to tracheal intubation during the course of the anaesthetic. In a recent series of patients undergoing parathyroidectomy, ventilation through a laryngeal mask airway was employed. The conversion rate to tracheal intubation was around 1% in overweight subjects and 7.2% in morbidly obese patients.

Consequently, the majority of patients require endotracheal intubation. This means that on the majority of occasions, the anaesthetist is faced with transition from anaesthesia involving controlled ventilation and endotracheal intubation to the fully awake state. This is potentially stormy. Clinically, the least desirable situation is the semi awake patient who has inadequate respiratory drive or airway reflexes to control respiration spontaneously, but who has sufficient reflexes to bite on the endotracheal tube, exacerbated by intermittent coughing or breath holding. In this situation, rapid basal collapse, atelectasis, and arterial desaturation occur. Removal of the endotracheal tube worsens the situation, as neither patient nor doctor has control of the airway. Equally, leaving the endotracheal tube in position may be problematic, because of ongoing airway stimulation and hypoxaemia. This can lead to a vicious circle of events, where re-sedation is employed to gain control. The scene is then set for a repeat of the entire cycle.

To avoid problems of this nature, the anaesthetic technique deployed should be consistent with rapid emergence from anaesthesia and good early airway control. Additionally, such techniques have the theoretical advantage of producing less post-operative respiratory depression, and therefore facilitating earlier discharge from a high dependency area. There has been intense interest in anaesthetic pharmacology in recent years, leading to the development of a number of 'clean' short acting agents which are suitable for the morbidly obese.

Particular interest has focused on desflurane, sevoflurane, propofol, and remifentanil. Studies of these agents have included traditional 'head-to-head' comparisons, as well more subtle studies where measures of depth of anaesthesia are used, rather than comparison of theoretically equipotent doses.

In an early study, Juvin and colleagues compared the recovery profiles of desflurane, propofol, and isoflurane following anaesthesia for gastric banding. In their study, anaesthesia was induced by propofol target controlled infusion, which was then continued throughout the case in the propofol group, but discontinued and substituted with either desflurane or isoflurane in the other groups. Muscle relaxation was facilitated with rocuronium, and analgesia provided by a target controlled infusion of alfentanil. Interestingly, in this study, the investigators chose to supplement anaesthesia with nitrous oxide. Depth of anaesthesia was monitored using bispectral index.

The study showed a marked difference in recovery profile between the three agents, with desflurane performing significantly better than the other two. Differences in quality of recovery could still be detected 2 h after the end of anaesthesia (see Figure 10.1).

Recently, interest has focused on differences in stability during anaesthesia and recovery profile between the two modern volatile agents, desflurane and sevoflurane. Where these are administered by a bispectral index controlled system, using the 'inhalational bolus' technique, both agents perform well as clinical anaesthetics during obesity surgery. Sevoflurane is associated with tighter control of

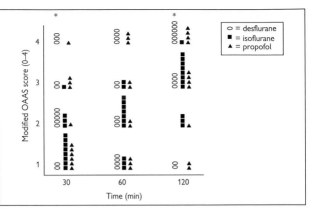

Figure 10.1 Observer's assessment of alertness/sedation (OAAS) score following isoflurane, propofol, and desflurane anaesthesia. A significant difference is seen between the desflurane group and the propofol and isoflurane groups. Reproduced from Juvin et al. (2000), Postoperative recovery after desflurane, propofol, or isoflurane anesthesia among morbidly obese patients. *Anesth Analg* **91**(3): 714–19, with permission from the International Anesthesia Research Society (IARS) and Lippincott, Williams & Wilkins.

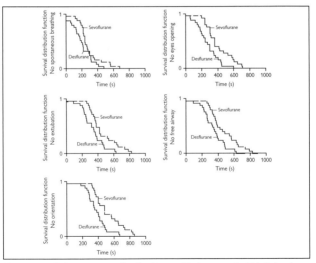

Figure 10.2 Early recovery profile after bispectral index controlled inhalational bolus techniques for desflurane and sevoflurane, showing 'survival curves' for different measures of recovery. Reproduced from De Baerdemaeker et al. (2003), Optimization of desflurane administration in morbidly obese patients. *Br J Anaesth* **91**(5): 638–50, with permission from Oxford University Press and the British Journal of Anaesthesia.

a bispectral index, and desflurane anaesthesia with fewer episodes of hypotension. Measures of early recovery suggest more rapid emergence from anaesthesia and improvement in psychometric and motor function in desflurane treated patients (Figure 10.2). However, these differences are of borderline clinical significance. Nausea seems to be of shorter duration in sevoflurane-treated patients, and there are no clinically important differences in post-operative hypoxia or discharge times from the post-operative anaesthetic care unit.

Several investigators have looked at the use of nitrous oxide during laparoscopic bariatric surgery. Nitrous oxide is associated with a rapid profile of recovery. Although it is has been claimed that nitrous oxide leads to bowel distension and poor operating conditions, in a randomised controlled trial, there was no clinically detectable difference in operating conditions between patients anaesthetised with or without nitrous oxide supplementation.

Further improvements in recovery profile have been made possible by target controlled remifentanil infusion. Although this leads to a more rapid emergence from anaesthesia, it is also associated with problems with early post-operative pain control. Clinically, pre-emptive analgesia is required prior to discontinuation of the remifentanil infusion to avoid development of 'rebound' pain.

10.2 Post-operative analgesia

Many strategies have been employed for post-operative anaesthesia in the morbidly obese. This has been intensively studied in the bariatric surgery population as well as other patient groups undergoing both laparotomy and peripheral surgery.

In the immediate post-operative period, patients undergoing bariatric surgery are treated according to a multimodal approach. This includes a combination of paracetamol, non-steroidal anti-inflammatory drugs [cyclo-oxygenase (COX) 1 and 2] together with opioid analgesics.

Data from the psychological literature suggest that patients undergoing bariatric surgery have reduced analgesic requirements compared with others. This may reflect a high degree of patient motivation in individuals undergoing bariatric surgery, or may be a more general reflection of changes in the behaviour and function of central opioid receptors in obesity (see Chapter 2).

Following either open or laparoscopic bariatric surgery, effective analgesia can be provided by the combination of non-specific non-steroidal anti-inflammatory drugs (COX 1 and 2 inhibitors) together with a parenteral opiate. Patient controlled morphine is frequently employed for this purpose. The use of non-steroidal anti-inflammatory drugs helps reduce the total opioid requirement. However, the effect on respiratory depression remains uncertain.

This risk of obstructive sleep apnoea or the obesity hypoventilation syndrome persists for several days, and is not limited solely to the period of anaesthesia or opioid infusion. This is because both anaesthesia and opioids alter the nature of sleep, and suppress periods of deep and REM sleep. Following recovery from the effects of sedative drugs – commonly on the third or fourth post-operative night – there is a rebound in the proportion of REM sleep. This can in extreme cases increase to around 80% of the total sleep period. The increase in REM sleep is associated with obstructive sleep apnoea and disordered respiratory control, and so in the recovery 'rebound' period, patients continue to be at increased risk of nocturnal hypoxaemia. This in part accounts for the well-known observation that perioperative myocardial ischaemia occurs most commonly on the second and third post-operative nights.

Traditional (COX 1 and 2) non-steroidal anti-inflammatory drugs can be supplemented by paracetamol (acetominophen). Although the precise actions of paracetamol remain unknown, many of its actions have been attributed to a central COX 3 effect. Paracetamol can be given orally, rectally, or parentally. Since the recent introduction of intravenous paracetamol, its use for acute perioperative pain has increased dramatically. It is a very valuable clinical adjunct for perioperative pain management in the morbidly obese. Because it is distributed largely to the central compartment, the dose used in the morbidly obese patients is similar to that used in non-obese subjects (in absolute terms). An increase in the size of the dose could lead to toxicity. However, as there is increased clearance of paracetamol in obesity, the dosing frequency may need to be increased. Some anaesthetists suggest that morbidly obese patients should be given a 1 g bolus five times daily in the immediate perioperative period.

10.3 **Regional anaesthesia**

A number of regional anaesthetic techniques can be used either as sole therapy for post-operative pain or as an adjunct. The choice of block and technique depends on the nature and site of surgery. For minor and body surface procedures, local infiltration may prove sufficient.

Specific nerve blocks and plexus blocks are best performed under ultrasound control. Basic bedside ultrasound machines designed for vascular access are inadequate, as they give insufficient resolution at depth. More sophisticated equipments, such as those found in the radiology department, can give excellent images and result in safe and highly successful nerve and plexus blocks. Ultrasound has proved particularly valuable when attempting to block the brachial plexus by the subclavicular approach, and for sciatic nerve block.

Following open bariatric surgery or other midline laparotomy, much of the pain experienced relates to the trauma of access. Good quality pain relief is achieved by a combination of patient controlled analgesia with poly-modal non-steroidal anti-inflammatory therapy. This can be supplemented by a rectus abdominis sheath block. The rectus sheath block can be performed by the surgeon under direct vision, or by the anaesthetist under ultrasound control. 20 mL of 0.5% bubivacaine are infiltrated into the medial border of each of the rectus abdominis muscles. The local anaesthetic spreads upwards and downwards through the muscle from the point of injection, and gives post-operative analgesia improved early post-operative analgesia how can the time when analgesic requirements greatest. The effects on the post-operative oxygenation and respiratory function are not known.

10.4 **Central neuraxial blockade**

Both spinal and epidural blocks have been performed for conduct of anaesthesia and post-operative pain relief in the morbidly obese. Even when used for lower abdominal surgery, subarachnoid block produces more severe deterioration in respiratory function in the morbidly obese compared with non-obese subjects. This persists into the post-operative period. However, the deterioration in respiratory function in patients operated under spinal anaesthesia is less than that observed following general anaesthesia.

Similar results have been observed with epidural anaesthesia. Thoracic epidural anaesthesia has often been advocated for use in the morbidly obese undergoing upper abdominal surgery. It is technically difficult to site a thoracic epidural catheter in the morbidly obese patient, and there is a relatively high failure rate compared with non-obese subjects. However, this should not preclude thoracic epidural analgesia in high-risk cases. Many benefits have been claimed for thoracic epidural anaesthesia, including a reduced risk of thromboembolic complications and improved post-operative respiratory function.

Compared with post-operative opioid analgesia, there is better respiratory function and preservation of vital capacity whether thoracic epidural technique is used (Figure 10.3). Therefore, patients with significant respiratory disease undergoing major abdominal surgery may benefit from elective placement of a thoracic epidural catheter.

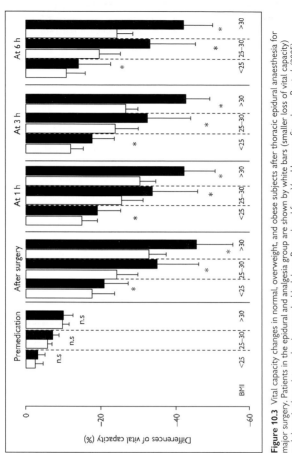

Figure 10.3 Vital capacity changes in normal, overweight, and obese subjects after thoracic epidural anaesthesia for major surgery. Patients in the epidural and analgesia group are shown by white bars (smaller loss of vital capacity) and those in the opiate analgesia group by black bars. Reproduced from Von Ungern – Sternberg, B. et al. (2005). Comparison of perioperative spirometric data following spinal or general anaesthesia in normal-weight and overweight gynaecological patients. *Acta Anaesthesiol Scand* **49**(7): 940–8, with kind permission of Blackwell Publishing.

However, excellent results have been achieved after bariatric surgery by use of more conservative measures. Consequently, the choice of analgesic method should be carefully considered, taking into account both the likely risk benefit ratio to the patient, the likelihood of success, the skill and usual practice of the anaesthetist, and three facilities available for post-operative monitoring and care.

10.5 **Post-operative fluid management**

Post-operative fluids should be administered with an awareness of the changes in patient physiology seen following obesity. Fluid management depends on the fluid balance of the individual patient. Specific fluid losses relating to the surgical procedure as well as insensible losses must be replaced. Baseline fluid requirements and insensible losses are related to body surface area.

The situation is additionally complicated in many patients by the presence of diabetes. This may mandate administration of a glucose-containing infusion to support an insulin sliding scale regimen. Because many obese patients suffer from type 2 diabetes with insulin resistance, they have a relatively low risk of diabetic ketoacidosis. Fluid management involving minimal glucose supplementation (predominantly based on administration of a balanced salt solution) can be clinically highly effective.

The presence of right heart failure or cor pulmonale (often associated with either left heart failure or peripheral oedema) should alert the clinician to the potential need for fluid restriction. In this situation, early reinstitution of habitual diuretic therapy helps to maintain appropriate fluid balance. Central venous pressure monitoring and regular weighing are also useful strategies to aid management of fluid balance.

Following surgery, many patients become oliguric not because of central volume fluid depletion, but rather because of the neurohumoral stress response. The syndrome of inappropriate antidiuretic hormone secretion should be suspected on the basis of a high urinary osmolarity combined with a low plasma osmolarity. Treatment options include fluid restriction or administration of a very small dose of a loop diuretic – often, this results in a spectacular diuresis.

10.6 **Recovery environment**

Post-operatively, morbidly obese patients should be nursed an appropriate environment. Depending on the presence or absence of co-morbidities and the magnitude of surgery, this can range from a short stay in a recovery unit followed by discharge home, to an overnight stay in a post anaesthetic care unit, or admission to a high dependency or intensive care bed.

In general, morbidly obese patients with significant co-morbidity undergoing body cavity surgery should, at a minimum, remain in a 24-h post anaesthetic care unit or high dependency unit. This environment allows continuous monitoring of cardiovascular variables and oxygen saturation. Facilities should be available not only for supplemental oxygen, but also for CPAP, chest physiotherapy, and nebulisers. At the end of the initial 24-h period in the post anaesthetic care unit, a decision is taken, based on the patient's clinical progress, as to whether it is appropriate to step care down to ward-based care. If this is inappropriate, the patient can be transferred to an intensive care unit for further management. If no appropriate post-operative care facility is available, elective surgery should not proceed.

10.7 **Conclusions**

Effective post-operative analgesia, fluid management, and respiratory care can be provided in a range of environments. In practice, however, this usually means a prolonged stay in a post anaesthetic care unit or a high dependency unit. A multimodality approach to pain management helps limits the maximum dose of any one particular class of agent. This is important, as morbidly obese patients suffer a range of co-morbidities which places them at increased risk of drug-related complications. The patient's habitual medications should be reinstituted as soon as possible following surgery. This may require adjustment of the dose or the route of administration.

Further reading

Arain SR, Barth CD, Shankar H, Ebert TJ (2005). Choice of volatile anesthetic for the morbidly obese patient: sevoflurane or desflurane. *J Clin Anesth* **17**(6): 413–19.

De Baerdemaeker LE, Struys MM, Jacobs S, Den Blauwen NM, Bossuyt GR, Pattyn P, Mortier EP (2003). Optimization of desflurane administration in morbidly obese patients: a comparison with sevoflurane using an 'inhalation bolus' technique. *Br J Anaesth* **91**(5): 638–50.

De Baerdemaeker LE, Jacobs S, Den Blauwen NM, Pattyn P, Herregods LL, Mortier EP, Struys MM (2006). Postoperative results after desflurane or sevoflurane combined with remifentanil in morbidly obese patients. *Obes Surg* **16**(6): 728–33.

Juvin P, Vadam C, Malek L, Dupont H, Marmuse JP, Desmonts JM (2000). Postoperative recovery after desflurane, propofol, or isoflurane anesthesia among morbidly obese patients: a prospective, randomized study. *Anesth Analg* **91**(3): 714–19.

Norman J, Aronson K (2007). Outpatient parathyroid surgery and the differences seen in the morbidly obese. *Otolaryngol Head Neck Surg* **136**(2): 282–6.

Strum EM, Szenohradszki J, Kaufman WA, Anthone GJ, Manz IL, Lumb PD (2004). Emergence and recovery characteristics of desflurane versus sevoflurane in morbidly obese adult surgical patients: a prospective, randomized study. *Anesth Analg* **99**(6): 1848–53.

von Ungern-Sternberg BS, Regli A, Reber A, Schneider MC (2005). Effect of obesity and thoracic epidural analgesia on perioperative spirometry. *Br J Anaesth* **94**(1): 121–7.

von Ungern-Sternberg BS, Regli A, Reber A, Schneider MC (2005). Comparison of perioperative spirometric data following spinal or general anaesthesia in normal-weight and overweight gynaecological patients. *Acta Anaesthesiol Scand* **49**(7): 940–8.

Chapter 11

Bariatric surgery and post-operative outcome

> **Key points**
>
> - Outcomes following anaesthesia and surgery in the morbidly obese are reasonably good.
> - Several large reported series have failed to confirm body mass index as an independent risk factor for adverse outcome.
> - Poor outcome is related to the presence of co-morbidities.
> - Patients undergoing open surgery have been shown to develop higher post-operative into abdominal pressures than those undergoing similar surgical procedures laparoscopically.
> - Three principles underlying bariatric surgery are reduction in stomach size, gastric outlet restriction, and malabsorption.
> - Early surgical procedures such as jejunoileal bypass had an unacceptably high post-operative complication rate.
> - Current surgical procedures include laparoscopic adjustable gastric banding and gastric bypass Roux loop reconstruction.
> - These techniques have a relatively low complication rate.
> - There is a clearly demonstrable effect of programs size, with larger programs having better outcomes.

Anaesthesia for the morbidly obese is challenging, partly because of technical challenges, but largely because of the co-morbidities suffered by this patient population. In a survey published by Royal College of Anaesthetists (London), over 50% of critical incidents (many of which were near misses) reported obesity as a factor. Outcomes following anaesthesia and surgery in this patient group have however been reasonably good. Several large series have failed to confirm body mass index as an independent risk factor for adverse outcome. Rather, poor outcome is related to the presence of co-morbidities, but not more so than in a non-obese population with the same co-morbidities. Absolute numbers of adverse outcomes are greater in the morbidly obese because of their higher prevalence of co-morbidity, not because of high body mass index.

There are two major exceptions to this general rule. The first of these relates to intra-operative surgical complications, which have a higher incidence in the morbidly obese as compared with the general population. Second, there is a higher incidence of post-operative nosocomial infections in the morbidly obese.

Surprisingly, despite the finding in functional clotting studies (thromboelastogram and Sonoclot) that the morbidly obese are hypercoagulable, there is a surprisingly low incidence of clinically detectable deep vein thrombosis (in one study, around 0.25%). Such studies are a largely retrospective. Several authors have suggested that the absence of relatively low rate of adverse outcomes reflects greater clinical care being exercised when looking after the morbidly obese.

Equally, in the day case setting, morbidly obese patients do not have a worse outcome than non-obese subjects, based on the body mass index alone. Absolute complication rates reflect the fact that co-morbidities are encountered more commonly in the morbidly obese population than in their lean counterparts.

Post-operative nausea and vomiting are a major problem following surgery in the obese. After laparoscopic bariatric surgery, around two-thirds of patients experience nausea and vomiting in the recovery room. Although anti-emetics are effective, one of the more interesting factors to have a major independent effect on post-operative nausea and vomiting is intra-operative fluid administration. Patients receiving larger volumes of fluids, particularly when administered rapidly, are less likely to suffer post-operative nausea and vomiting.

Patients undergoing open surgery develop higher post-operative intra-abdominal pressures than those undergoing similar surgical procedures laparoscopically. Open surgery patients have, correlated with this, a greater post-operative fluid requirement and a poorer urine output. The abdominal compartment syndrome has been proposed as a major cause of post-operative renal dysfunction in morbidly obese patients undergoing major surgery.

11.1 **Bariatric surgery**

Many strategies have been used in the treatment of severe obesity. These include combinations of diet, behavioural therapy, and drug treatment. Many patients find even aggressive therapy ineffective in the long term. Typically, they experience cycles of weight loss and regain, often with overshoot (yo-yo phenomenon). Patients who have repeatedly failed to lose weight in a sustained fashion with conservative measures should be considered for bariatric surgery. Bariatric surgery, for many, offers the only proven means of achieving long-term weight reduction. It is also effective in reducing obesity-related co-morbidities. Bariatric surgery has been endorsed as a beneficial and cost-effective health care intervention by consensus guidelines in many countries. In the United States, its role has been well established since the National Institutes of Health 1991 guidelines. In England and Wales, it is endorsed by NICE guidelines, and in Scotland, by SIGN guidelines. Similar guidelines exist throughout Western Europe.

Bariatric surgical procedures are based around three principles. The first involves reduction in stomach size. This is achieved by mechanical means so that food enters a small upper gastric pouch before passing either into the lower part of the stomach or into the intestine. Early filling of the upper part of the stomach (the pouch) means that it is difficult or uncomfortable for the patient to eat large volumes quickly.

The second bariatric surgical principle involves restriction of the size of the gastric outlet. This means that, once the stomach or gastric pouch has been filled, it remains full for a prolonged period of time.

The third principle involves induction of malabsorption, usually by intestinal bypass.

A frequently observed consequence of bariatric surgery is that patients rapidly lose hunger while eating. This may be due to anatomical changes in the stomach, or early passage of food into the intestine. Following gastric bypass surgery many patients experience early satiety associated with increased protein YY_{3-36} (satiety hormone) and greater blunting of ghrelin (hunger hormone) levels, as compared with gastric banding and normal controls. Consequently, gastric bypass patients develop a rapid indifference to further food. Changes in these and other gut hormones are thought to influence responsiveness of insulin receptors, and play a role in the rapid resolution of type 2 diabetes seen following gastric bypass surgery.

11.2 **Outcomes after bariatric surgery**

A number of weight reduction surgical procedures have been practised. Through the 1960s and first half of the 1970s, a commonly performed operation was the jejunoileal bypass. This proved popular as a means of producing rapid, effective, and sustained weight loss. In this operation, the proximal jejunum was anastomosed to the distal ileum, 10 cm before the caecum. This resulted in a very short length of functional bowel available for absorption of nutrients, together with a long blind loop.

However, it was associated with a number of post-operative complications which limited its usefulness. The most severe early complication was acute liver failure. This was seen in around 7% of patients. A number of patients also went on to develop hepatic fibrosis. This can occur even in the late post-operative period. Its prevalence and severity increase with time after surgery. There are several reports of patients requiring liver transplantation following jejunoileal bypass.

Organ-specific problems were also seen in other systems. Rapid weight loss, and in particular, protein loss, resulted in cardiac failure in some patients. The formation of kidney stones was also a common problem, occurring in around one-third of patients in most series.

Other problems seen after jejunoileal bypass, and after some more modern operations, include malabsorption and dumping. Malabsorption syndromes following bariatric surgery are related to which parts of the small intestine are bypassed, and how much is bypassed. Consequently, malabsorption following jejunoileal bypass has the potential to be severe.

There is loss of absorption of vitamins from the duodenum and jejunum. Reduced absorption of calcium and iron are common following all forms of bariatric surgery, but are particularly severe after jejunoileal bypass. Long-term vitamin B12 supplementation was almost invariably required after jejunoileal bypass, and maybe required (either parentally or sub-lingually) after gastric bypass surgery. Following other forms of bariatric surgery, it can be a problem because of the reduced functional volume of the stomach, resulting in reduction in intrinsic factor and the secondary failure to absorb vitamin B12 despite an intact intestine. Malabsorption of other B group vitamins, particularly thiamine, is also seen after many variants of bariatric surgery.

The 'dumping' syndrome results from excessively rapid passage of food, particularly sugary foods, into the small intestine. Patients experience pallor, sweating, and dizziness, often accompanied by a sensation of doom. They may have to lie down for half an hour or so until the unpleasant sensation passes. These unpleasant symptoms are frequently followed by diarrhoea.

In the first few months following jejunoileal bypass, and for a variable period of time after that, there were significant problems with ongoing diarrhoea and electrolyte disturbances including hypokalaemia and dehydration. The problems following jejunoileal bypass were so severe both physiologically and symptomatically that around one-third of patients subsequently underwent reversal of their surgery. About 11–12% of patients died more than 30 days after jejunoileal bypass. Two-thirds of the patients died before bypass reversal, 13%

at the time the reversal, and a further 23% after reversal. Not surprisingly, jejunoileal bypass is seldom offered nowadays.

The second traditional operation, still practised, is 'stomach stapling' or vertically banded gastroplasty. In this operation, the stomach is divided into a small upper segment and a larger lower portion. These communicate through a narrow opening. Consequently, eating is rapidly followed by a sensation of satiety. Food passes more slowly into the lower part of the stomach. This type of procedure does not induce malabsorption, and while it is successful in some patients, it is of limited value in producing sustained long-term weight loss. The upper part of the stomach may distend over time, and the banding line disrupts, allowing full communication between the two parts of the stomach. Adverse effects of malabsorption are not a feature of this operation, although oesophageal reflux and 'productive burping' are unpleasant for the patient.

Nowadays, the most common pure restrictive operation is adjustable gastric banding. This is generally performed laparoscopically. In this operation, a band is placed around the upper part of the stomach, dividing it into a small upper pouch of around 25 mL, and a larger lower segment. This is essentially a restrictive procedure. The band is adjusted by injection saline into a subcutaneous reservoir. By this means, over a period of weeks, the band can be progressively tightened until the patient reaches a point where early satiety and weight loss can be balanced against unpleasant side effects. For this device to be successful, considerable compliance is required from the patient together with intensive follow-up. Some patients continue to overeat, and the upper gastric pouch becomes distended so that early satiety no longer prevents overeating. In some patients, the band can become displaced. The adjustable gastric band is extremely popular, and is particularly successful in patients at the lower end of the morbid obesity range. An alternative to laparoscopic banding is sleeve gastrectomy, which can also be performed laparoscopically. In this operation, the volume of the stomach is reduced, but without outflow obstruction. This results in early fullness, but not malabsorption.

Probably the most popular and successful operation for patients at the upper end of the morbid obesity range, and moving into the super obese range, is the 'gastric bypass' (Figure 11.1).

This operation involves a staple line across the upper stomach to reduce gastric volume 2 between 25 and 40 mL. This is combined with a Roux loop reconstruction, inducing partial malabsorption. The anastomosis between the upper gastric pouch (neo-stomach) and the Roux loop is small, so as to introduce a restrictive element to the operation. The procedure has two main variants, based on a short or a long Roux limb. The Roux loop effectively prevents reflux and ulceration, but potentially can induce malabsorption in some patients, although not invariably. Therefore, long-term dietary supplementation is advisable. Severe malabsorption and dumping are uncommon.

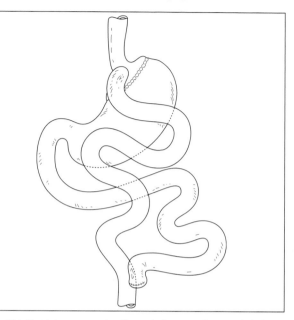

Figure 11.1 Gastric bypass operation. The staple line across the stomach divides it into a small upper pouch (neo-stomach) and a larger residual gastric remnant. Both gastric components are joined to intestine, the large gastric remnant by its original duodenal connection, and the neo-stomach by a Roux loop.

A similar operation is the so-called duodenal switch. In this operation, a long limb intestinal bypass carries foods to the distal small bowel. Bile and pancreatic juices are carried in a second, shorter limb. These two limbs join together, so that the common limb in which digestion and absorption occur together is very limited.

The malabsorption operations share the complications of the jejunoileal bypass, though to a much lesser degree. These are seldom severe or life threatening. Ultimately, all forms of bariatric surgery are reversible, though this is very rarely required in clinical practice. Mortality following gastric bypass surgery has been estimated at between 0.25 and 1%. There is a clearly demonstrable effect of programs size, with larger programs having better outcomes and lower mortality rates than small programs. American data have suggested that there is a very steep learning curve, with the majority of complications occurring in the first 100 cases performed by each surgeon.

This has led, in the United States, to the development of a list of recognised 'centres of excellence' for bariatric surgery. Although formal lists of 'centres of excellence' are not available in Europe, the centre effect still applies.

11.3 Beneficial outcomes of bariatric surgery

The majority of patients undergoing bariatric surgery (predominantly either laparoscopic banding or one of the variants of gastric bypass surgery) achieve successful, sustained weight loss over a period of months. World Health Organisation guidelines suggest that the maximum weight change should not exceed 0.5–1 kg per week. Weight loss more rapid than this is likely to lead to muscle loss and cardiac problems.

Depending on the precise operation performed, weight loss continues until the patient is around 10–20% above their ideal body weight. It 'levels off' at this value, as energy intake and expenditure are now in balance. Very few patients overshoot to a weight below their ideal body weight. Where this does occur (e.g., following extensive malabsorption procedures such as the jejunoileal bypass), high protein and calorie supplementation are ineffective at remedying the problem. A surgical solution may be required.

Diabetes resolves very rapidly and generally long before weight loss has been achieved. Indeed, this has led some surgeons to perform gastric bypass surgery in non-obese diabetic patients in an attempt to modify their diabetes.

As weight loss progresses, fatty infiltration around the airway is lost early on. This leads to a rapid resolution of obstructive sleep apnoea and obesity hypoventilation syndrome. Other conditions such as asthma also resolve relatively early in the weight loss process. Resolution of hypertension may take a little longer, and may not be permanent. The majority of patients observe dramatic improvement in other symptoms, particularly arthritic symptoms in the hips, and knees and ankles, and psychological problems (see Figures 11.2 and 11.3).

Overall, the majority of patients undergoing bariatric surgery are extremely satisfied with the result in terms of improvement in general health and resolution of co-morbidities. Many forms of cosmetic surgery can be justified on health economic and quality grounds in terms of their beneficial effects on psychological co-morbidity and improvement in body image. Although bariatric surgery is not performed for cosmetic reasons, many patients experience improvement in body image and derive consequent lifestyle benefits that have wide reaching general health implications.

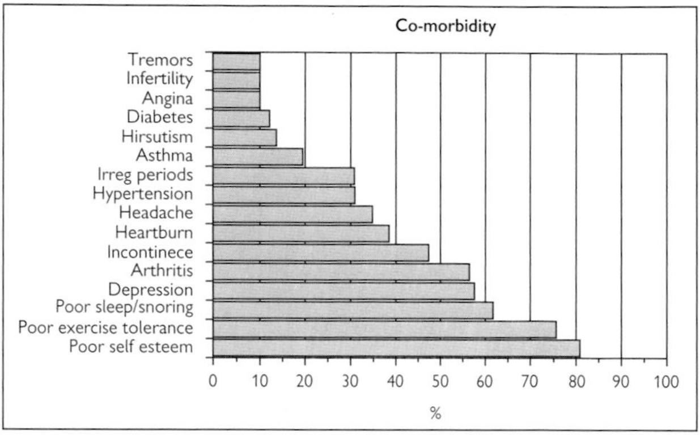

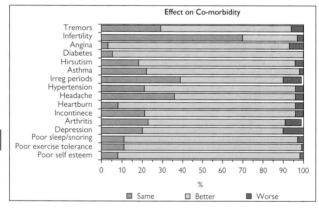

Figure 11.2 Prevalence of obesity related co-morbidities (data from 305 consecutive patients undergoing gastric bypass surgery). Courtesy of Mr Stephen Pollard, consultant surgeon, Leeds

Figure 11.3 Change in patients' perception of co-morbidities following gastric bypass surgery. Courtesy of Mr Stephen Pollard, consultant surgeon, Leeds

Further reading

Dindo D, Muller MK, Weber M, Clavien PA (2003). Obesity in general elective surgery. *Lancet* **361**(9374): 2032–5.

Forrest JB, Rehder K, Cahalan MK, Goldsmith CH (1992). Multicenter study of general anesthesia. III. Predictors of severe perioperative adverse outcomes. *Anesthesiology* **76**(1): 3–15.

Gonzalez QH, Tishler DS, Plata-Munoz JJ, Bondora A, Vickers SM, Leath T, Clements RH (2004). Incidence of clinically evident deep venous thrombosis after laparoscopic Roux-en-Y gastric bypass. *Surg Endosc* **18**(7): 1082–4.

Klasen J, Junger A, Hartmann B, Jost A, Benson M, Virabjan T, Hempelmann G (2004). Increased body mass index and peri-operative risk in patients undergoing non-cardiac surgery. *Obes Surg* **14**(2): 275–81.

Nguyen NT, Lee SL, Anderson JT, Palmer LS, Canet F, Wolfe BM (2001). Evaluation of intra-abdominal pressure after laparoscopic and open gastric bypass. *Obes Surg* **11**(1): 40–5.

Pivalizza EG, Pivalizza PJ, Weavind LM (1997). Perioperative thromboelastography and sonoclot analysis in morbidly obese patients. *Can J Anaesth* **44**(9): 942–5.

Schuster R, Alami RS, Curet MJ, Paulraj N, Morton JM, Brodsky JB, Brock-Utne JG, Lemmens HJ (2006). Intra-operative fluid volume influences postoperative nausea and vomiting after laparoscopic gastric bypass surgery. *Obes Surg* **16**(7): 848–51.

Index